ESSENTIALS OF NEUROCHEMISTRY

Gaynor C. Wild

Edward C. Benzel

University of New Mexico, Albuquerque

Jones and Bartlett Publishers

Boston   *London*

Editorial, Sales, and Customer Service Offices
Jones and Bartlett Publishers
One Exeter Plaza
Boston, MA 02116
1-800-832-0034
617-859-3900

Jones and Bartlett Publishers International
PO Box 1498
London W6 7RS
England

Library of Congress Cataloging-in-Publication Data

Wild, Gaynor C.
    Essentials of neurochemistry / Gaynor C. Wild, Edward C. Benzel.
      p. cm.
    Includes bibliographical references and index.
    ISBN 0-86720-862-7
    1. Neurochemistry. I. Benzel, Edward C. II. Title.
    [DNLM: 1. Neurons—physiology—programmed instruction.
  2. Neuroregulators—physiology—programmed instruction.
  3. Receptors, Neurotransmitter—physiology—programmed instruction.
  4. Nervous System Diseases—physiopathology—programmed instruction.
  WL 18 W668e 1994]
  QP356.3.W54 1994
  612.8′042—dc20
  DNLM/DLC
  for Library of Congress   93-47356
                                                CIP

Printed in the United States of America
98 97 96 95 94   10 9 8 7 6 5 4 3 2 1

CONTENTS

PART TWO
SYNAPSES AND TRANSMITTERS   31

Chapter 3 • The Synapse   33

Chapter 4 • Amino Acid Neurotransmitters   44

Chapter 5 • Acetylcholine   54

PART THREE
RECEPTORS   87

PART FOUR
ORGAN NEUROCHEMISTRY   117

Chapter 12 • Learning and Memory   119

Chapter 13 • Addiction and Receptor Regulation   130

Chapter 14 • Brain Energy Metabolism   143

PART FIVE
MEDICAL NEUROCHEMISTRY   155

Chapter 15 • Acid–Base Balance and CNS Injury   157

PREFACE

This book is an outgrowth of teaching neurochemistry to first-year medical students, senior undergraduate students, and beginning graduate students. Its aim is to provide an introduction to the principles of neurochemistry, building upon the basics of biochemistry. Some background in biochemistry and biology is assumed, but we have tried to base our discussions on the working knowledge that introductory courses provide.

Our focus throughout the text is on integration, both between neurochemistry and biochemistry and between neurochemistry and the other neurosciences. We have also striven throughout for clarity, at the expense of encyclopedic coverage; i.e., we have tried to keep the book small, concise, and digestible. This approach necessitates the omission of many interesting and thought-provoking subjects. The most difficult decisions for us have been what not to include.

Research in neurobiology, including neurochemistry, is advancing at a very rapid pace. The 1990s has been designated the "Decade of the Brain," and every issue of major journals announces important new advances. It is especially challenging to attempt to write a text on a topic that is changing so rapidly. This is yet another reason for focusing on basic principles and sacrificing some detail. We hope we have chosen wisely.

To facilitate readability, the text is arranged into parts, each with a specific theme:

Part One, Structural Neurochemistry
Part Two, Synapses and Transmitters
Part Three, Receptors
Part Four, Organ Neurochemistry
Part Five, Medical Neurochemistry

This arrangement enables those who wish to focus on a specific segment of neurochemistry to do so.

In writing this book, we have benefited greatly from advice and discussion with colleagues, most particularly Mark Bitensky and Margaret Whalen. Most of all, we have benefited from the comments and advice of students and house officers. We are indebted to these people; without their contributions, this work would not have been possible.

Structural Neurochemistry

CHAPTER 1

Central Nervous System Cell Types

NEURONS

Although the brain is considered to be a single organ, its internal structure and organization are quite complex. Viewed as a whole, it contains about 10^{11} neurons, arranged in many groupings, called **nuclei,** that are more or less related by function. These nuclei, consisting of neurons and their supportive material, constitute the gray matter of the **central nervous system (CNS).**

Neurons vary considerably in size and shape, but have important biochemical and physiological properties in common (Figure 1-1). Neurons are excitable, being able to generate the electrical activity called action potentials. Each neuron usually contains an axon (a long process leading from the cell body to another cell) and can propagate action potentials along the full length of the axon—even when the axon is several feet in length. The majority of axons within the CNS, however, are only a centimeter or two in length. Within the CNS, most axons make functional connections with other neurons at junctions called synapses. Synapses may be located on the cell body of another neuron (**axo-somatic** synapses), but most are thought to contact dendrites (Figure 1-1) (**axo-dendritic** synapses). Less commonly, synapses allow contact between one cell's axon and another cell's axon (**axo-axonic**, or presynaptic, synapses).

Other types of cellular communication also occur in the brain, through mechanisms such as dendro-dendritic contacts and the release of transmitter from non-synaptic sites. The greatest attention, however, has been paid to axo-dendritic synapses, which are the paradigm example.

Once neural cells differentiate into mature neurons, they lose their ability for mitosis. This means that fully differentiated, post-mitotic cells cannot be replaced during the lifetime of the organism. As neurons die in the course of normal aging, they cannot be replaced. Therefore, the maximum number of neurons exists near the time of birth. The "normal" loss of neurons has been estimated to be about 10^3 per hour, although this figure has recently been questioned. In the average lifetime of about 75 years (660,000 hours), this would constitute a loss of only 0.66 percent of the total number of neurons present at birth. People of advanced age do, in fact, have noticeably less brain substance than their younger counterparts. It is possible, however, that brain shrinkage with age could be due to decreasing size of neurons, rather than to their loss. In addition,

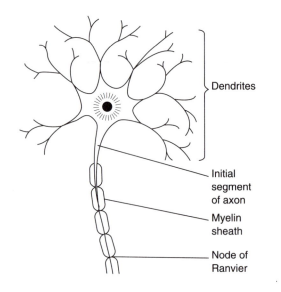

Dendrites

Initial segment of axon

Myelin sheath

Node of Ranvier

Figure 1-1 Diagram of a Nerve Cell and Its Processes

various aspects of one's environment, from accidents to drug use, can increase the rate of either cell shrinkage or cell loss.

GLIA

Although neurons are thought of as the primary cells of the nervous system, there are large numbers of other cells, called glia. The term "glia" comes from "glue," which portrays a simplistic view of their function by early neuroanatomists. Glial cells are only about one-tenth the size of neurons. Since the number of glial cells is ten times greater than that of neurons in the brain (approximately 10^{11} neurons and 10^{12} glial cells), the glia constitute approximately half of the overall mass of the brain. The areas of brain called **white matter** consist predominantly of glial cells and a small volume of axons.

There are three types of glia: astrocytes, oligodendrocytes, and microglia. They arise from two different embryological lines. Microglia are derived from mesoderm, whereas all other brain cells are derived from ectoderm.

Astrocytes

Astrocytes, which nearly completely surround every neuron's plasma membrane (Figure 1-2), also surround all cerebral blood vessels. This fact has led to the belief that astrocytes may, in fact, constitute the **blood–brain barrier.** Unlike neurons, astrocytes retain the ability for mitosis. They therefore form the equivalent of scar tissue in brain. They proliferate in areas of traumatic or degenerative neuronal cell loss. Astrocytes and microglia may be the only cells in the brain that retain mitotic capability throughout the lifetime of the individual. Astrocytes also can depolarize, much as neurons do, but much more slowly. Astrocytes, however, are not excitable (i.e., an action potential does not develop). Their depolarization takes place over seconds, but an action potential is over in hundreds of milliseconds.

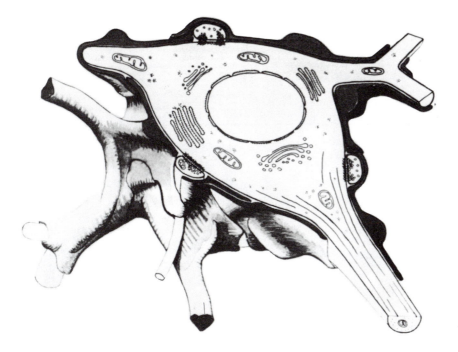

**Figure 1-2
Diagrammatic
representation of the
relationship between a
neuron and astrocytic
processes.** *The surface
of the neuronal soma is
covered with thin
cytoplasmic extensions
of astrocytes. These also
ensheath synaptic
regions. In the more
distal regions of the
dendrite, groups of
synaptic terminals are
often surrounded by a
common astrocytic
mantle.*

Astrocytes appear to have a specific, "reciprocal" metabolic relationship with their neighboring neurons. When neurons are excited, they rise to a higher level of electrical activity and their metabolic rate increases. During this excitation, nearby astrocytes decrease their energy demands. The astrocytes recover later, after the neurons have returned to their baseline level of metabolic activity.

There is also evidence for a substantial biochemical intimacy between astrocytes and neurons, including the transfer of macromolecules from astrocytes to neurons. Claims have been made for the transfer of fully formed RNA and protein molecules, although the mechanisms by which such transfers could occur are not clear. In any event, astrocytes and neurons are closely associated, both anatomically and metabolically. This close association appears to be of importance for CNS function.

Oligodendrocytes

Oligodendrocytes are the source of CNS **myelin** (discussed in the following section; see Figure 1-3). Like neurons, oligodendrocytes probably do not retain the capacity for mitosis. A single oligodendrocyte may provide a portion of myelin to as many as fifty or more different axons (Figure 1-4). This anatomical relationship would appear to preclude the retention of mitotic ability, as the involvement of axons and their associated myelin segments is so intimate and mutually dependent. The survival of either cell directly depends on the other.

Microglia

Microglia may not arise embryologically from the same ectodermal source as other neural cells, and, in fact, may enter the brain continuously from the blood.

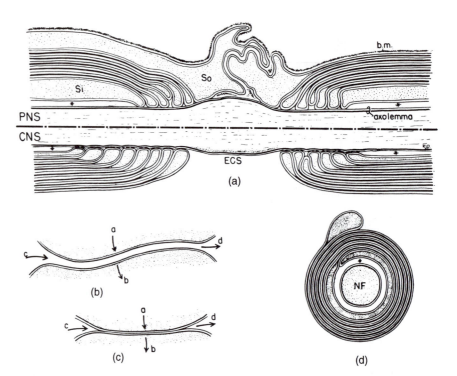

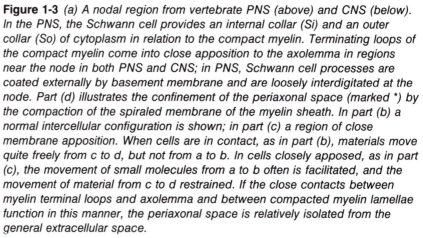

Figure 1-3 *(a) A nodal region from vertebrate PNS (above) and CNS (below). In the PNS, the Schwann cell provides an internal collar (Si) and an outer collar (So) of cytoplasm in relation to the compact myelin. Terminating loops of the compact myelin come into close apposition to the axolemma in regions near the node in both PNS and CNS; in PNS, Schwann cell processes are coated externally by basement membrane and are loosely interdigitated at the node. Part (d) illustrates the confinement of the periaxonal space (marked *) by the compaction of the spiraled membrane of the myelin sheath. In part (b) a normal intercellular configuration is shown; in part (c) a region of close membrane apposition. When cells are in contact, as in part (b), materials move quite freely from c to d, but not from a to b. In cells closely apposed, as in part (c), the movement of small molecules from a to b often is facilitated, and the movement of material from c to d restrained. If the close contacts between myelin terminal loops and axolemma and between compacted myelin lamellae function in this manner, the periaxonal space is relatively isolated from the general extracellular space.*

They function within the CNS as brain macrophages (i.e., scavengers that destroy foreign matter and digest the debris) and may play a significant role in immunological diseases of brain, including **autoimmune** diseases. If microglia do, in fact, enter the brain from the blood on a continuous basis, a significant modification of the traditional concept of the blood–brain barrier is in order. Traditionally, the blood–brain barrier was thought not to allow the passage of whole cells. These assumptions have been challenged by many recent observations, including even the direct observation, by electron microscopy, of **leukocytes** appearing to penetrate the lining of cerebral blood vessels.

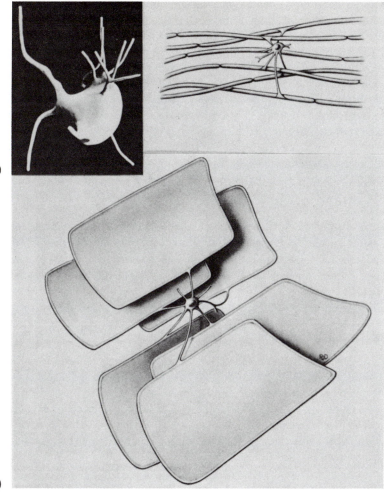

(c)

(a)

(b)

Figure 1-4 Drawings to show the CNS myelin-related cell (the oligodendrocyte) and its postulated relation to segments of myelin. *(a) The configuration of the cell body as reconstructed from serial sections (from Stensaas and Stensaas, 1968). (b) The oligodendrocyte in continuity with many segments of myelin in the usual spiraled and compacted configuration. (c) The myelin segments in an unrolled configuration. The cytoplasmic extensions of the oligodendrocyte related to myelin have certain similarities to the axonal extensions of neurons.*

MYELIN

Myelin is the name given to the multi-layered spiral of oligodendrocyte membrane that surrounds axons. Each myelin segment originates from a single oligodendrocyte. Each oligodendrocyte contributes many myelin segments, but each segment is apparently associated with axons from different neurons. This anatomical arrangement, which is not found in the **peripheral nervous system (PNS),** creates one possible mechanism for a kind of chemical integration among neurons. That is, if glial cells can pass molecules to neurons, then a single oligodendrocyte could pass molecules to each of the dozens of different neurons it myelinates. This mechanism could contribute to the integration of the functions of these associated neurons.

Characteristics of Myelination

Myelination occurs predominantly just prior to and/or following birth, depending on the species. In general, the more mature an organism is at the time of birth, the greater the extent of myelination. In humans, myelination occurs predominantly after birth, with the majority taking place during the first two years of life.

The sequence of myelination corresponds roughly to **phylogenesis,** or the evolutionary sequence. The peripheral nervous system (PNS) myelinates first, followed by the spinal cord. The cerebral cortex and the rest of the forebrain myelinate much later. Arcuate fibers, which connect different portions of the cerebral cortex to each other, are the last to be myelinated. Although it is experimentally difficult to determine when myelination is complete, because of practical difficulties in measuring a process's ending, arcuate fibers probably are not completely invested with myelin until the third decade of life. This essentially coincides with the appearance of the last wisdom teeth, and may indicate that biological maturity is only achieved after about two and a half decades in humans.

The myelin investment around an axon is functionally beneficial. As its myelination increases, the neuron is capable of increasing its rate of firing. Similarly, increasing the rate of excitation of neurons in a developing brain increases the rate of myelination. The two processes, therefore, drive each other and are interdependent.

Benefits of Myelin

The fundamental basis of the distinctions between myelinated and unmyelinated fibers is not the presence of glial cells, as unmyelinated fibers also are surrounded by oligodendrocytes, but the presence of the myelin sheath (Figure 1-3). Myelinated axons need only have action potentials at the nodes of Ranvier, the unmyelinated sections of membrane, which are up to 1 mm apart. Action potentials are not propagated in each successive increment of membrane, as they must be in unmyelinated fibers. This process, of the action potential's moving from node to node rather than continuously, is called **saltatory** conduction.

The myelin sheath serves to optimize the function of the neuron in at least three ways (listed below in order of increasing importance). First, myelin serves as an electrical insulator. In demyelinating diseases, the loss of this insulation results in an electrical "cross talk" between adjacent axons, which can be pathologically disruptive to brain function. Second, myelin increases conduction velocity. Finally, myelin decreases the metabolic demand necessary for the generation of an action potential.

The velocity of a conducted action potential in a myelinated axon is directly proportional to the diameter of the axon plus the myelin sheath. Unmyelinated axons (which are still surrounded by glial cell bodies, but not by multi-layered myelin sheaths) have been observed to conduct action potentials in direct proportion to the square root of the axon's diameter. This distinction is of considerable importance in the peripheral nervous system, as differently myelinated axons conduct at varying velocities. There are, however, a large number of axons in the CNS that gain little conduction velocity from myelination. For axons of very small diameter (in the range of 0.2 μm), myelination does not provide a conduction velocity advantage, as the resistance to conduction is high in volumes of cytoplasm this small. Many axons in the CNS approach this diameter.

From a metabolic point of view, myelinated fibers have a three-hundred to four-hundredfold advantage over non-myelinated fibers with respect to their energy needs. Because action potentials need be generated only at nodes, the amount of energy necessary to restore normal ion balances across the membrane of the axon after the action potential has passed is reduced. An unmyelinated fiber must restore ionic gradients along the entire length of its axonal membrane.

The Molecular Architecture of Myelin

Since the myelin sheath is composed of multiple layers of compacted plasma membranes, it contains the same molecules as the membranes of other cell types in addition to characteristic myelin molecules. Certain myelin-specific molecules are of considerable interest, both in terms of their unique functions regarding myelin and because of their potential contribution to disease processes. Although myelin traditionally was thought of as being metabolically inert, its molecules are now known to turn over at a significant rate. In addition, some of its unique molecules function as autoantigens, and thereby can play a role in the development of CNS diseases.

Cholesterol. The most abundant molecule in myelin, on a molar basis, is **cholesterol** (Figure 1-5). In this regard, myelin is similar to membranes in other cells, except that CNS cholesterol is predominantly unesterified. Most cholesterol in other animal membranes has a fatty acid attached to its hydroxyl group by an **ester** linkage. This linkage is similar to that by which fatty acids are attached in phospholipids, triacylglycerols, etc. Esterified cholesterol, however, is found in significant quantities in the CNS in certain pathological states. In the demyelinated lesions of multiple sclerosis, for example, the percentage of esterified cholesterol is significantly increased.

Phospholipids. The predominant phospholipid in myelin is phosphatidyl ethanolamine (PE) (Figure 1-5). This fact is peculiar to brain tissue, as phosphatidyl choline (PC) is the major phospholipid in other tissues. Most phospholipids, as indeed nearly all lipids, contain fatty acid **residues.** There are a few lipids, however, that contain **alkyl** chains, physically similar to fatty acids, but at a different level of oxidation. Therefore, these residues are not fatty acids, but fatty **aldehydes** or **alcohols.** These less common structures are more common in brain than in other tissues, and this is especially true of PE. The PE of brain contains a large percentage of molecules, called plasmalogens, of which one of the chains yields an aldehyde, rather than an acid.

This subgroup contains a fatty acid in ester linkage at the second position of the glycerol, but has an **ether** group at the first position. The ether can contain a **saturated** carbon chain, making it an alkyl ether; more commonly, the chain in the ether linkage has one or more double bonds. If a double bond occurs between the first and second carbon, the chain behaves as an aldehyde. The double bond in this location rearranges upon **hydrolysis,** yielding a long-chain aldehyde, rather than a fatty acid. Because of this susceptibility to hydrolysis, which is lacking in alkyl ethers, plasmalogens may have functional roles distinct from those of alkyl ethers or diacyl ester phospholipids. These roles are yet to be fully characterized.

Sphingolipids. (See Chapter 2 for more detailed discussion.) Another peculiarity of brain tissue is the large amount of sphingolipids it contains. This is true both

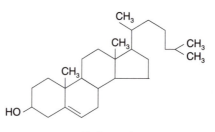

Cholesterol

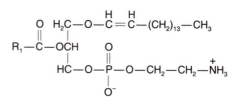

A phosphatidyl choline (PC)

Figure 1-5 Molecules
of Myelin

A plasmalogen of phosphatidyl ethanolamine (PE)

of white-matter myelin and of gray matter (neurons and their surroundings). Sphingolipids, by definition, contain a residue of **sphingosine,** which is a long-chain fatty base. They also contain a fatty acid attached in **amide** linkage to the second carbon of the sphingosine. This molecule of sphingosine plus a fatty acid is called a **ceramide.** It does not itself appear in significant quantities in nerve tissue, but it is an obligatory metabolic intermediate for all sphingolipids.

The sphingolipids of myelin are simpler in structure than those of neurons. Most have only one or two residues attached to the ceramide. The first carbon of the sphingosine chain is most commonly linked to a residue of galactose in myelin. A minority of myelin sphingolipids are also phospholipids, with a phosphoryl **choline moiety** linked as a diester to carbon 1. This latter molecule is called **sphingomyelin,** which is a somewhat misleading name, as sphingomyelin actually occurs in all mammalian membranes. Sphingomyelin was discovered in brain white matter, and was named after it.

The three-dimensional structure of sphingomyelin gives it considerable resemblance to phosphatidyl choline (PC). Indeed, the two lipids can be hydrolyzed by some of the same enzymes. Furthermore, sphingomyelin and PC are both localized to the outer leaflets of plasma membranes.

The most characteristic lipid of myelin is another sphingolipid, **cerebroside,** in which the substituent on the first carbon of the ceramide is galactose. Large amounts of cerebroside are present in myelin, and much of this is synthesized after the blood–brain barrier has formed. This fact, which is also true of many other brain molecules, implies that the body's immune system does not fully recognize cerebrosides (and these other molecules) as "self," and therefore is capable of mounting an immune response to them. That is, if cerebrosides or similar autoantigens appear in the bloodstream, the body can mount an immunological attack against them. Under ordinary circumstances, of course, cerebroside does not appear in blood, as it turns over completely within the white matter of the CNS, sequestered from the immune system by the blood–brain barrier.

A derivative of cerebroside, called sulfatide, contains a sulfate residue on the 3′ hydroxyl group of the galactose of the cerebroside. This molecule also occurs characteristically in myelin. Sulfatides have a negative charge, from the sulfate group. Another derivative of cerebroside, with some characteristics similar to those of sulfatide, occurs when cerebroside has a **sialic acid** residue (also named N-acetyl neuraminic acid, or NANA) attached to the same 3′ position. This molecule, called **ganglioside** GM4, also has a negative charge, as a result of the sialic acid.

GM4 is an unusual ganglioside in that the **sugar** attached to the ceramide is not glucose. The majority of gangliosides contain glucose in this position, as will be discussed in Chapter 2. GM4 is like other gangliosides, however, in that its sialic acid residue is attached to a galactose. The only other ganglioside found in significant quantities in myelin is ganglioside GM1. GM1, in common with all other gangliosides of the CNS, is found in neurons. Since it is also present in myelin, it is not specific to either white or gray matter.

Sphingomyelin is not peculiar to brain, and may therefore be recognized as "self" by the immune system. Many negatively charged molecules, and especially negatively charged lipids, do not serve well as antigens. This may be due to the fact that many self molecules are negatively charged, and immune responses against them are suppressed in the process of the body's learning to recognize self. These facts may help explain why the major lipid **autoantigen** of myelin appears to be cerebroside. That is, if myelin, or crude white matter, is injected into another animal of the same species, it will initiate the production of antibodies and sensitized immune cells. This will occur even if the myelin is injected into an identical twin of the animal from which the molecules were taken. Some of these immune responses are specific for myelin proteins, but some are specific for cerebroside. Therefore, cerebroside is one of the immunologically "characteristic" molecules of myelin.

Proteins. Among the proteins of myelin are several that are specific to white matter. These also can function as autoantigens. The two major such molecules are myelin basic protein (MBP) and proteolipid protein (PLP). MBP, often thought of as the major autoantigen of white matter, is not an integral membrane protein, but is found in the soluble cytoplasmic compartment of the oligodendrocyte.

Immune Properties of Myelin Molecules. Like myelin basic protein (MBP), the proteolipid protein (PLP) is peculiar to myelin and is predominantly synthesized after the blood–brain barrier has sequestered the CNS from immune surveillance. PLP is a highly unusual protein in many ways, and it is quite different from MBP. PLP is an **integral** membrane protein, spanning the membrane in which it occurs. It has some structural features in common with neurotransmitter receptors, which also span membranes, but it is not known to have a receptor function. Its most unusual structural feature is that fatty acids are attached to the protein, as esters. This modification results in the protein's having many lipid-like properties and fewer protein-like properties than would be expected from its **amino acid** composition. For example, PLP is soluble in organic solvents, such as chloroform, and is not soluble in water. PLP also has autoantigenic properties.

MBP alone, when injected into another organism of the same species, generates an immune response. In fact, MBP can be used experimentally to generate an autoimmune disease called experimental autoimmune encephalomy-elitis (EAE). EAE is considered by many to be an animal model for multiple sclerosis (MS). However, EAE, when produced solely by the use of MBP, differs from multiple sclerosis in many respects, principally in that EAE does not wax and wane as MS does. Thus, there has been considerable effort to create animal models with more of the clinical features of MS. Several recent models use a mixture of autoantigenic molecules. Such autoimmune "cocktails" usually include MBP, cerebroside, PLP, and often a ganglioside. Although such cocktails can produce a CNS white-matter disease with many features of MS, questions about the appropriateness of the models remain. Indeed, some experts question the validity of the theory of an autoimmune mechanism as a cause of MS.

AXOPLASMIC TRANSPORT

As mentioned, axons connect neuronal cell bodies to synaptic terminals and may be quite long (up to several feet, in some cases). Most are myelinated on the outside, with the plasma membrane, called the axolemma, exposed only at nodes between the myelin segments. These nodes are called the nodes of Ranvier. Inside the axon, in addition to the normal cytoplasm found in a cell, there is considerable molecular architecture, called the cytoskeleton. The cytoskeleton is composed of an array of proteins, variously connected among themselves, and consisting of three general classes: microfilaments, intermediate filaments, and microtubules. There are many different types of proteins incorporated into these structures, but the major one is tubulin, polymers of which form the basis of microtubules. Tubulin is a major protein in neurons, because of its high concentration in axons and other neuronal processes.

Microtubules can be properly thought of as the major structure within axons, but they are not contiguous throughout the length of the axon. They were originally assumed to form a continuous structure, analogous to railroad tracks, from the **perikaryon** to the synaptic terminal. More recent research has shown that microtubular structures are actually fairly short, much less than 1 mm in length, and that they overlap. The only cellular structure that may in fact be continuous throughout the axon is the smooth **endoplasmic reticulum.**

It is now clear that there is considerable two-way traffic through an axon, with large quantities of cellular materials of various kinds continuously being transported in both directions at once. Transport that moves in the same direction as the action potential, from the cell body to the synaptic terminals, is known as anterograde transport. This type of transport is usually divided into two large subcategories: fast and slow. Slow axonal transport is further subdivided into two rates: a few mm per day, called SCb, and a few tenths of a mm per day, called SCa. SCb is most likely similar to the "cytoplasmic streaming" observed in hepatocytes and other cells. SCb is the rate at which molecules found in the soluble cytoplasm, such as the enzymes of glycolysis, move. SCa is the speed at which parts of the cytoskeleton, such as neurofilaments and microtubules, move down the axon. The SCa rate is so slow that it requires months for substances to travel the length of an average axon within the CNS. Slow transport has recently been shown to require energy, although the amount required is not high.

Fast anterograde transport, which also has subdivisions, requires both an intact cytoskeleton and mitochondria (for the production of ATP). The rate of fast transport is in the range of hundreds of mm per day and it allows replacement of components of the synaptic terminal every few hours, or even every few minutes, in the case of shorter axons. Fast transport requires energy in the form of ATP, and it moves cellular organelles, such as mitochondria and lysosomes. Fast transport also appears to move the material from which synaptic vesicles are made. It operates continuously, as long as there is an energy supply. Different particles move at different rates, presumably because of the stops and starts involved with moving from one microtubular structure to another.

There is also a retrograde transport mechanism, in the direction from the synaptic terminal to the cell body (or perikaryon). Retrograde transport is also fast (i.e., about 100 mm per day) and consists predominantly of the cellular organelles called **lysosomes** and their contents. Lysosomes, each of which is enclosed by a membrane, are found throughout neural cells. They contain only hydrolytic enzymes, and, as a rule, have the ability to hydrolyze all of the macromolecules in the cell. Lysosomes may also play a role in secretion, and are known to be involved in the continuous recycling of neurotransmitters and their associated cellular elements (see Chapter 3). A significant fraction of this recycled material is returned to the cell body by retrograde transport, apparently in, or accompanying, lysosomes.

The existence of axonal transport systems and the fact that the fast systems require an intact cytoskeleton and a continuous supply of ATP were known long before the specific molecules, or "motors," that power the systems were discovered. Four such motors are now known, one of which, myosin, is devoted to muscle contraction. Two others, kinesin and dynein, both occur in axons and are involved in fast flow. The fourth, dynamin, also occurs in neurons and is involved in slow transport.

Kinesin is usually thought of as the motor for anterograde movement and dynein as the motor for retrograde movement. Both molecules are associated with microtubules. Microtubules are enormous polymers of tubulin. Tubulin can be purified in such a way that it retains the directionality it has in vivo. Both kinesin and dynein have been studied in vitro, where it is possible to observe their movement along such polarized tubulin fibers. In an in vitro system, each molecule moves only in one direction along the tubulin. Kinesin moves toward the "plus," or synaptic, terminal end; dynein moves toward the "minus" end, in the direction of the cell body. Both molecules use the energy of hydrolysis of ATP (although kinesin appears to be able to use GTP as well) to move both themselves and the substances to which they bind. The movement, at least in the case of kinesin, is rather like that of an inchworm, with the protein reversibly folding up into a U and then stretching back out.

Dynamin, the more recently discovered motor involved in slow flow, also uses energy, in the form of GTP. It took longer to discover this, apparently because of both the slowness of the turnover and the fact that ATP is not the preferred source of energy. Dynamin appears to move the cytoskeleton itself, in reference to another bit of cytoskeleton. The net forward movement can be quite slow.

SELF-STUDY QUESTIONS

Facts:

1. What are the anatomical relationships between glia and neurons?

2. What are the differences between glia and neurons in number, metabolism, capability for mitosis, and size?

3. Describe the sequence of myelination, and relate it to evolution.

4. Describe three ways in which myelin has evolutionary utility to the operation of the nervous system.

5. Describe the patterns of myelination in the central nervous system (CNS) and the peripheral nervous system (PNS). Describe the ratio of axons to glia and glia to neurons.

6. What are phospholipids? cerebrosides? sulfatides? cholesterol?

7. What are the autoantigens of myelin?

8. Describe three different kinds of axoplasmic flow, in terms of direction, relative velocity, and substances moved.

Concepts:

1. Describe two possible mechanisms by which an autoimmune disease of the CNS could arise.

2. Discuss the relationship between neuronal function and myelination.

3. Discuss the reciprocal relationship between neuronal and glial metabolism, and its possible role in the function of the CNS.

4. Discuss the possible significance of the transfer of large molecules from glial cells to neurons.

5. Describe the benefits of myelin to the cell.

BIBLIOGRAPHY

Bunge, R.P. 1970. Structure and function of neuroglia: Some recent observations. In *The Neurosciences: Second Study Program,* edited by G.C. Quarton, T. Melnechuck, and G. Adelman. New York: Rockefeller University Press.

Morell, P., Quarles, R.H., and Norton, W.T. 1989. Formation, structure, and biochemistry of myelin. In *Basic Neurochemistry,* edited by G. Siegel, B. Agranoff, R.W. Albers, and P. Molinoff. New York: Raven Press.

Quarles, R.H., Morell, P., and McFarlin, D.E. 1989. Diseases involving myelin. In *Basic Neurochemistry,* edited by G. Siegel, B. Agranoff, R.W. Albers, and P. Molinoff. New York: Raven Press.

Vallee, R.B., and Bloom, G.S. 1991. Mechanisms of fast and slow axonal transport. *Annual Review of Neuroscience* 14: 59–92.

CHAPTER 2

Brain Sphingolipids

STRUCTURE OF SPHINGOLIPIDS

As noted in Chapter 1, sphingolipids contain a long-chain fatty base, called sphingosine, and a fatty acid attached in amide linkage to the second carbon of the sphingosine. This combination of fatty acid and sphingosine is called ceramide (Figure 2-1). Sphingosine, by definition, is the central feature of all sphingolipids. With the exception of sphingomyelin (which is a choline-containing phospholipid, as well as a sphingolipid), sphingolipids contain sugars, making them also **glycolipids,** or glycosphingolipids (GSLs). The first sugar residue is attached to the terminal OH group of the sphingosine, the second sugar is attached to the first, and so on.

Sphingosine contains two **hydroxyl** groups, an **amino** group, and a *trans* double bond, in addition to the alkyl chain. Sphingosine was discovered by J.L.W. Thudichum in the latter nineteenth century. Thudichum named sphingosine after the sphinx, because he thought it would not yield its secrets. Indeed, the secrets of sphingolipid function(s) remain closely held: none of the role(s) of sphingolipids in brain function are clear today.

Sphingosine is synthesized from palmitoyl CoA and the amino acid serine. The **hydrophobic** end (the thirteen-carbon chain in Figure 2-1) comes from the palmitoyl group, and the **hydrophilic** end (with a nitrogen and two oxygens) comes from serine. The synthetic reaction requires **pyridoxal phosphate,** as it involves decarboxylation of an amino acid. The double bond is added by an enzyme after the **saturated** molecule, called sphinganine, is synthesized.

The significance of the *trans* double bond, unusual in alkyl groups in biology, is unknown. *Trans* double bonds do not, in general, change the overall shape of a molecule very much, giving it a three-dimensional structure very similar to that of a comparable molecule without double bonds.

In the absence of pathology, some of which is discussed later, the amino group of sphingosine is in amide linkage with a fatty acid, making a ceramide. Free sphingosines and free ceramides are not normally found in living tissue in significant quantity, as both molecules serve only as metabolic intermediates. Complete glycosphingolipids contain hydrophilic groups of varying sizes and character, attached to the OH group of the number 1 carbon of the ceramide.

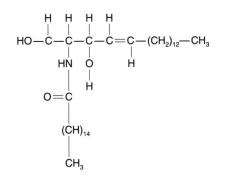

Figure 2-1 A ceramide.
The example shown here consists of palmitic acid attached to the most common sphingosine, containing eighteen carbons and a trans double bond.

Sphingolipids are **polydisperse,** in that their structures are variable; there is variation even in the structure of a single, "pure" lipid molecule. For example, a ceramide with a single sugar attached to the first carbon is called a cerebroside (Figure 2-2). Purification of the cerebroside from normal brain white matter yields a molecule that contains only galactose as the sugar. It is therefore considered to be pure galacto-cerebroside. However, the sphingosine shown in Figure 2-1, with one double bond and eighteen carbons, is not the only sphingosine. Some sphingosines have no double bonds and others have different numbers of carbons (twenty, twenty-two, and higher). In addition, the ceramide portion of the molecule can contain any one of several different, naturally occurring fatty acids. Thus, a "pure" cerebroside is in fact a family of closely related molecules, not a single molecule. This aspect of structure is called "polydisperse" and is found in all lipids and in most carbohydrate-containing molecules. These kinds of molecules are thus much more variable in structure than nucleic acids or proteins.

The fatty acid in glycosphingolipids (GSLs) varies, and there are relatively characteristic patterns of fatty acids associated with different hydrophilic groups and with different cells of origin. The more complex gangliosides (see below) are made in neurons and contain about 90 percent stearic acid (C18:0). (This notation, C18:0, indicates that stearic acid is a fatty acid with eighteen carbons and no

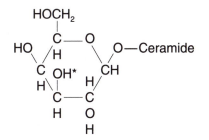

Figure 2-2 A galacto-cerebroside.
The asterisk indicates the site of attachment of either a sulfate residue, making a sulfatide, or a sialic acid residue, making ganglioside GM4.

double bonds.) Cerebrosides, synthesized in oligodendrocytes, contain a biphasic distribution of fatty acids, with large amounts of palmitic acid (C16:0) and of fatty acids with twenty-four carbons. The longer fatty acids can be saturated (for example, lignoceric acid, C24:0) or **unsaturated** (nervonic acid, C24:1); a fraction even has a hydroxyl group on the number 2 carbon (cerebronic acid, C24:0).

The characteristic fatty acid pattern sometimes makes it possible to determine the cells of origin of sphingolipids found in remote locations. For example, brain is the likely source of the sphingolipid that accumulates in the spleen in Gaucher's disease. This is indicated by the fact that the sphingolipid in such cases contains predominantly stearic acid, similar to gangliosides.

The simple saccharides in sphingolipids (in descending order based on their approximate quantities in whole brain) are galactose, glucose, N-acetyl galactosamine, N-acetyl glucosamine, fucose, and inositol. Other carbohydrates can be found in trace quantities. Many different patterns of carbohydrate structure are found. Most brain GSLs, however, contain one of only five or six different sets or patterns of carbohydrates.

The majority of white-matter GSLs have only a single carbohydrate residue, galactose. Gray-matter GSLs are more complex, but many of them are based on a single carbohydrate sequence, containing only four sugars in the carbohydrate core. A common sequence found in the GSLs of neurons is glucose, galactose, N-acetyl galactosamine, galactose. The glucose residue is attached to the ceramide, a characteristic of neurons.

The incorporation of sialic acid (also called N-acetyl neuraminic acid, or NANA) in a GSL characterizes it as a ganglioside. Sialic acid (Figure 2-3) is a complex, nine-carbon sugar containing a **carboxyl** group at carbon 1, which usually has a negative charge. It is a **ketose** (as the glycosidic linkage is made to carbon 2) and an amino sugar. (The amino group contains an N-acetyl group on carbon 5.) In vivo, it is usually attached either to a galactose residue or to another sialic acid. Sialic acid is found in the outer carbohydrate layer of all cells, being attached both to glycoproteins (at terminal positions) and to gangliosides. The total number of sialic acid residues on the surface of a cell contributes to many aspects of its function, including contact inhibition and possibly the specificity of binding to small molecules.

Figure 2-3 Sialic Acid (N-Acetyl Neuraminic Acid)

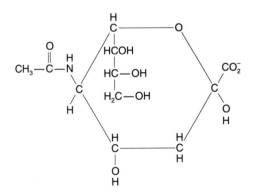

ANABOLISM OF GLYCOSPHINGOLIPIDS

Addition of a sugar to a ceramide creates a glycosphingolipid (GSL). This usually occurs in the Golgi apparatus of the cell. The nature and sequence of sugar residues that are added to the growing lipid are specific for different types of neural cells. Galactose is attached directly to the ceramide in oligodendrocytes, and glucose is most commonly attached to the ceramide in neurons. A ceramide with only a galactose added is a cerebroside, and is one of the immunologically characteristic and specific molecules in myelin (see Chapter 1). Cerebrosides can be further modified by attachment of either a sulfate residue or a sialic acid residue at the third carbon of the galactose. This creates a sulfatide or ganglioside GM4, respectively (Figure 2-2).

All the molecules mentioned above are found in myelin and are synthesized within oligodendrocytes. The actual attachment of a sugar residue (called **glycosylation**) is carried out by enzymes specific for the particular sugar and for the recipient ceramide. The glycosylation of proteins also occurs in the Golgi apparatus.

In neurons, the initial glycosylation is the addition of the first carbon of glucose to the ceramide at carbon number 1. After this, a galactose is most frequently added (in **beta** 1⟶ 4 linkage, the number 1 carbon of the galactose being attached to the number 4 carbon of the glucose). This creates a lactosyl ceramide, since the tandem sugar residues have the same structure found in the **disaccharide** lactose (milk sugar). Lactosyl ceramide is the starting point for the synthesis of most brain gangliosides, since most gangliosides are in neurons. Addition of a single sialic acid residue to the hydroxyl in position 3 of the galactose creates ganglioside GM3 (Figure 2-4).

The carbohydrate chain to which sialic acid residues are attached defines the ganglioside, and is indicated in the name. In GM3, G stands for ganglioside, M for monosialo, and 3 refers to the lactosyl group. (The number itself is arbitrary, and was assigned to the molecules before their structures were known.) Adding another sialic acid residue to the first one produces GD3 (where D stands for disialo). T stands for trisialo, Q for quatrosialo, and P for pentasialo. Gangliosides

Figure 2-4   Schematic Structures of Two Important Gangliosides

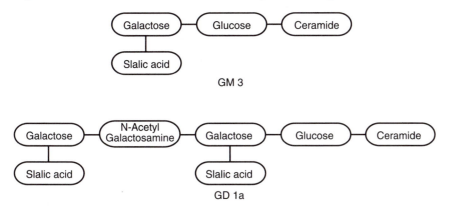

GM 3

GD 1a

GM3 and GD3 are the simplest, and are found in large concentrations only in certain tissues, such as those of the retina, the pineal gland, and some tumors. More commonly, a residue of N-acetyl galactosamine is added to position 4 of the galactose, creating GM2 (see Figure 2-5). A further addition of galactose, to position 3 of the N-acetyl galactosamine, creates GM1 (Figure 2-5), one of the most abundant gangliosides. The addition of another sialic acid residue to position 3 of the terminal galactose makes GD1a, the most abundant ganglioside in mammalian brain (Figure 2-4).

Larger and more complex gangliosides are, for the most part, made by adding residues of sialic acid or other carbohydrates to these fundamental

Figure 2-5   The Sequence of Enzymatic Degradation of GM1

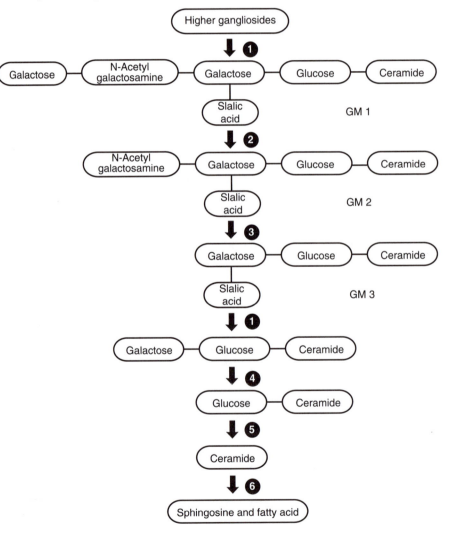

(See Table 2-1 for key to numbers representing enzymes.)

gangliosides. Inositol, fucose, and N-acetyl glucosamine are found in some gangliosides. Many sialic acid residues may be present on a single molecule. Gangliosides containing as many as five, six, or seven sialic acid molecules, with a total of as many as thirty sugars, are known.

Sialic acid is usually linked to the molecule at one of two points: either the 3' hydroxyl of a galactose or the 8 hydroxyl of another sialic acid. Since the number 1 carbon of sialic acid is an acid, the residue is attached to other sugars with its number 2 carbon, creating a glycosidic linkage. As a result, the carboxyl group is free, and thus is usually charged. Therefore, in most cases, the molecule containing sialic acid is negatively charged. Since sialic acid–containing lipids and proteins are found on the exterior surfaces of all cells, cells themselves are negatively charged. This fact probably explains the earlier observation that negatively charged molecules, especially glycolipids, are often not good antigens: the immune system's ability to recognize negative charges must be at least partially suppressed.

During GSL synthesis in the Golgi apparatus, each residue added to the growing glycolipid must come from an "activated" derivative. For thermodynamic reasons, two molecules (for example, a ceramide and a galactose) cannot simply be joined together to make a cerebroside. Most commonly, sugars are used to make glycolipids and other **glycoconjugates** from their uridine diphosphate (UDP) derivatives. This process is also seen, for example, in the synthesis of glycogen, where UDP-glucose is used. Unusual or special sugars, however, are added from other "activated" derivatives. Sialic acid is derived from cytidine monophosphate sialic acid (CMP-sialic), for example.

The enzymes that catalyze these stepwise additions, called glycosyl transferases, are relatively (but not totally) specific for both substrates. They place the appropriate sugar into the "correct" location in the growing lipid, but glycosyl transferases are not as specific as comparable enzymes that play a role in the synthesis of proteins or nucleic acids. Therefore, the frequency of "errors," or variability, in the products is much greater during synthesis of glycosphingolipids. This relative lack of specificity in the enzymes results in polydisperse, or microheterogeneous, products, to a much greater degree than does the synthesis of actual gene products (i.e., nucleic acids and proteins).

All known glycoconjugates, whether based on proteins or lipids, are membrane molecules, and so are transported from the Golgi to the membrane destination. Glycoconjugates occur in large quantities in the plasma membrane, the endoplasmic reticulum, and lysosomal membranes. The extent of glycosylation of many other cellular membranes is not yet well known.

CATABOLISM OF GLYCOSPHINGOLIPIDS

As mentioned, glycosphingolipids are membrane molecules, in common with other glycoconjugates. Neurons and oligodendrocytes, since they are postmitotic, remain in the organ until the death of the cell, when the turnover of all the molecules in the cell occurs. In the living cell, despite the fact that the cell must remain in place for a lifetime, there is a continuous metabolic turnover of all molecules, and of all parts of molecules. In the steady state, therefore, the rate of synthesis of any molecule must exactly equal its rate of degradation. If an imbalance between synthesis and degradation exists, either a buildup or a loss of the molecule will result. Most CNS molecules are continuously synthesized and broken down by organized systems of enzymes. These processes are regulated by normal metabolic controls. Most membrane molecules, as far as is known, are synthesized in the Golgi apparatus, transported to the membranes in which they function, and later broken down by **autophagy.** Autophagy (literally, "self-eating") is a lysosomal process, whereby portions of the cell, apparently chosen more or less at random, are engulfed into lysosomes, thereby creating secondary lysosomes, and their constituent molecules are hydrolyzed. Both the synthetic and catabolic processes for **glycoconjugate** metabolism are slow, and they occur in different parts of the cell.

Genetic Errors of Metabolism

An imbalance between synthesis and **catabolism** of membrane molecules will eventually result in either the loss of the molecule (and its function) or a buildup of the molecule. Accumulation (or storage) of many molecules results in toxicity by a variety of mechanisms. In the simplest cases, the toxicity may come simply from the excessive volume of stored material and its resulting physical interference with normal cellular processes. Deficiencies of synthetic enzymes or excessive activity of catabolic enzymes are rare, apparently because all CNS molecules are needed for normal growth, development, and function. Therefore, a mutation that causes a synthetic enzyme to be missing or deficient is usually lethal. Several defects of catabolism (i.e., CNS storage diseases) exist, however. A large fraction of genetically determined CNS storage diseases originate in the lysosomes. Table 2-1 summarizes the most common diseases caused by deficiencies of lysosomal enzymes for glycolipid catabolism. (The

Table 2-1 CNS Storage Diseases

	Enzyme	*Deficiency Disease*
1	Sialidase	Sialidosis
2	Beta galactosidase	GM1 gangliosidosis
3	Beta hexosaminidase	Tay–Sachs disease
4	Beta galactosidase	Lactosyl ceramidosis
5	Beta glucosidase	Gaucher's disease
6	Ceramidase	Farber's lipogranulomatosis
7	Sulfatase	Metachromatic leukodystrophy
8	Beta galactosidase	Globoid cell leukodystrophy (Krabbe's disease)
9	Sphingomyelinase	Niemann–Pick disease

number of each enzyme in Table 2-1 is used to identify that enzyme in Figures 2-5, 2-6, and 2-7.)

Continual, slow autophagy requires normal lysosomal function. The lysosomes, which contain only hydrolytic enzymes, digest the large molecules in the cell into smaller, non-hydrolyzable molecules. These digestion products—fatty acids, amino acids, individual **saccharides,** alcohols, and inorganic residues—are sometimes called "micromolecules," or the "building blocks" of biochemistry. After being freed by hydrolysis within the lysosome, these small molecules must leave the lysosomal lumen, usually by specific transporters, and reenter cellular pools. These small molecules can then be reused in synthesis, in this way recycling many times before actually leaving the cell or the CNS.

Deficiencies of Enzyme Activities

In the event of a deficiency in or the absence of a lysosomal enzyme, there may be no symptoms in the developing fetus. This is apparently because autophagy does not begin until after the intense period of synthetic activity during gestation and the immediate post-natal period. In several of the diseases discussed below, no symptoms are present at birth, even when there is a total absence of the enzyme's activity. Symptoms may appear as early as a few weeks to months after birth, when catabolism begins to play a major role and normal turnover rates should be established.

In several lysosomal storage diseases, there is a rough correlation between the degree of residual enzyme activity and the age of onset of symptoms. The more enzyme activity, the longer it takes for the toxic buildup of substrate and for symptoms to appear. In general, there is a safety factor in enzyme levels of about 50 percent, meaning that an individual with 50 percent of normal enzyme level is usually asymptomatic. Enzyme levels lower than 50 percent, especially enzyme levels as low as zero to 20 percent, usually result in symptoms, and often very severe ones. A complete lack of enzyme activity will produce symptoms in infancy, whereas a person with enzyme levels of 15 to 20 percent may not develop symptoms until adulthood.

The same kind of reasoning applies in both white- and gray-matter storage diseases. Given the size and heterogeneity of the human population, it can be assumed that any enzyme deficiency that is not lethal in utero does in fact appear in the population. This fact, coupled with the late development of catabolism of glycoconjugates mentioned above, allows a significant number of nervous system storage diseases to exist in any population; many of these diseases are invariably lethal, in time. Some of the most significant diseases, described in greater detail below, are invariably lethal within the first few months of life if the enzyme deficiency is complete.

SPHINGOLIPID STORAGE DISEASES OF GRAY MATTER

As mentioned, the membrane molecules of neurons apparently turn over only by autophagy, the slow process whereby the cell incorporates part of its own substance into its lysosomes. Other kinds of molecules within the cell can be catabolized by specific systems separate from lysosomes, but the membrane glycoconjugates appear to turn over only in lysosomes. Therefore, any disturbance of lysosomal function, either from environmental toxic processes or mutations, can produce a pathological imbalance.

Lysosomal enzymes are arranged in such a way that the sequence of hydrolysis is obligatory, at least for GSLs. Hydrolysis usually occurs in the reverse order from synthesis, starting at the outermost aspect of the carbohydrate moiety. Hydrolysis of gangliosides (the largest GSLs and the GSLs most characteristic of neurons) begins with the removal of their outermost sialic acid residues. These are removed by the enzyme **sialidase** (also called **neuraminidase**), which is found both in lysosomes and in cytoplasm. In cytoplasm, sialidase may be loosely associated with membranes. The lysosomal form(s) of sialidase are likely associated with the next enzyme in the sequence for hydrolyzing gangliosides, a beta galactosidase.

There are multiple forms of sialidase in lysosomes, including one for gangliosides and another for glycoproteins. The enzyme specific for gangliosides may not be associated with a deficiency disease, possibly because its absence is fatal. There is, however, a disease state involving a deficiency of the enzyme for glycoproteins, called sialidosis. Another rare disease, galactosialidosis, is caused not by a genetic deficiency of sialidase but by the absence of a protein that protects sialidase from being itself **digested** by a protease. Lacking the protective protein, both sialidase and its associated beta galactosidase are degraded, so the brain contains inadequate levels of both enzymes.

GD1a (Figure 2-4) and most of the other large, complex gangliosides are degraded to GM1 by sialidases. This means that GM1 is produced in significant quantity, as a metabolic intermediate in the breakdown of many other larger molecules. The catabolism of GM1 proceeds in a stepwise manner, starting with the terminal galactose. Figure 2-5 indicates this stepwise process.

If there is a deficiency of the enzyme responsible for the first step, beta galactosidase (#2 in Table 2-1), the result is a disease called GM1 generalized gangliosidosis. Both nervous system and peripheral involvement are observed in this disease. The normal degradation of glycoproteins in liver is also impaired, which results in an accumulation in the joints of unhydrolyzed carbohydrate sequences from glycoproteins. Major abnormalities occur in brain as well, since GM1 is also a substrate for the enzyme. Thus, GM1 accumulates. A child without enzyme activity appears normal at birth but will often display symptoms of developmental delay within two or three months. As the ganglioside accumulates in neurons, it aggregates, because of its hydrophobic character and its size. Each molecule, in addition to its size, carries a negative charge from the sialic acid, and is therefore unable to cross membranes. As a result, GM1 builds up in the lysosomes of the neuron. At autopsy, up to 90 percent of total brain weight may be made up of ganglioside. The engorged, enlarged lysosomes fill their neurons. This physically prevents brain function.

If beta galactosidase activity is normal, but there is a deficiency of the next enzyme in the sequence, Tay–Sachs disease results. A deficiency of this beta hexosaminidase (#3 in Table 2-1) (only one isozyme is usually absent) causes GM2 to accumulate. This is the most common human sphingolipid storage disorder. The gene frequency for Tay–Sachs disease is about 1 in 25 or 30 in Ashkenazi (Northern European) Jews, and about one-tenth of this frequency in all other groups. Heterozygotes, having about 50 percent of the normal amount of enzyme, are typically not affected. Couples who are both heterozygotes for this disease have a 25 percent chance of producing a homozygous child, who will have zero enzyme activity. The frequency of heterozygotes in the Ashkenazi Jewish community results in roughly a one-hundredfold increase in the incidence of the disease compared to other populations when both parents are of Ashkenazi background. The incidence is even higher than the above figures indicate in people whose ancestors came from particular portions of eastern Poland or western Russia.

No treatment is yet available for Tay–Sachs disease. Attempts have been made to treat lysosomal storage diseases in the periphery by administration of the missing enzyme, with some limited success. Gangliosidoses in the CNS are unaffected by this type of therapy because of the blood–brain barrier—lysosomal enzymes added to the blood do not successfully cross the blood–brain barrier. Similarly, lysosomal enzymes are not likely to be incorporated into the appropriate locations, even if injected directly in brain, because of their inability to cross cell membranes. At present, Tay–Sachs disease can be diagnosed in utero by measuring the enzyme levels in cells given off by the fetus, and the pregnancy can be terminated.

The next enzyme in sequence is sialidase (#1 in Table 2-1). Sialidase is not able to remove the sialic acid residue attached to the inner galactose of a ganglioside, as the position is too physically crowded (steric hindrance): the inner galactose residue has both a sialic acid and an N-acetyl galactosamine attached on adjacent carbons. The steric crowding that results from this inhibits the action of sialidase. The enzyme is free to act, however, after the removal of the amino sugar in sequence.

The product of this reaction is galactosyl glucosyl (i.e., lactosyl) ceramide; it is no longer charged, since it is not a ganglioside. Several different beta galactosidase deficiency states have been reported (#2, 4 and 8 in Table 2-1). Given that the deficiency disease states are separate, the beta galactosidases for cerebroside (see below), for the terminal galactose of GM1, and for the galactose of lactosyl ceramide must be different enzymes. When different enzymes catalyze the same reaction, they are called **isozymes.** The presence of two different isozymes for hydrolyzing galactose residues from GSLs in neurons may result from the physical organization of lysosomal hydrolases in a specific sequence.

Deficiencies of each of the remaining enzymes of ganglioside catabolism, beta galactosidase, beta glucosidase, and ceramidase, have been reported to cause storage diseases. The symptoms of these diseases, however, tend not to be as severe as those of the other diseases mentioned above. This difference in severity may be due, in part, to the physical properties of the molecules that are stored in each case. When the stored, undigested substrate is a charged molecule, it apparently is unable to cross the lysosomal membrane. This is despite the hydrophobic character of the remainder of the molecule. The stored molecule accumulates at the site of the hydrolysis, eventually causing brain damage "from the inside out." If the molecule is small enough, and uncharged, it may be able to cross membranes, leaving the lysosome and possibly the cell. In this case, the stored molecule may be able to enter the cerebrospinal fluid (CSF) and leave the CNS. This may be the case for deficiencies of enzymes 4, 5 and 6 in Table 2-1.

The flow of CSF from brain into blood is through a series of structures called arachnoid villi. One important aspect of flow through arachnoid villi is that it is bulk flow; i.e., molecules do not need to "cross" a membrane in the usual sense of moving through it. Whenever the fluid pressure is higher in the CSF than in the blood of the venous sinuses, fluid will flow down the pressure gradient without being filtered. This allows large molecules to leave the CNS and enter the general circulation. Molecules small enough to leave their cell of origin can then easily leave the CNS. This appears to be one of the reasons why storage diseases of many uncharged molecules have less severe symptoms than storage diseases of charged substrates. The uncharged molecule leaves the brain and may accumulate in tissue where it is less harmful.

For example, a deficiency of the beta glucosidase that removes the last sugar from a ganglioside allows the buildup of a ceramide with glucose attached. Gaucher's disease results. In this disease, the uncharged glucocerebroside accumulates mainly in the spleen, although its source is the ganglioside pool of neurons. The accumulation of this glycosphingolipid in the spleen is not, in most cases, associated with mental retardation. Compared to patients suffering from diseases involving the storage of charged molecules, such as Tay–Sachs disease, these patients have a much more benign condition.

SPHINGOLIPID STORAGE DISEASES OF MYELIN

White-matter glycoconjugates, like those in gray matter, appear to turn over only by autophagy. Again, the lysosomes involved in this process appear to be those of the cells that synthesized the molecules initially.

The enzymes of lysosomal catabolism in oligodendrocytes also appear to be physically and chemically organized within the organelle, resulting in a specific sequence of degradation. Again, the lysosomal catabolic sequence is the reverse of the synthetic sequence for sphingolipids. In white matter, this means that the initial step is the removal of any substituent on the galactose of the GSL, if one exists. Therefore, the sulfate residue or the sialic acid residue is the first to be hydrolyzed (see Figure 2-6). There is no evidence for a storage disease involving ganglioside GM4 in white matter, confirming the lethal character of an absence of sialidase in lipid catabolism.

A deficiency disease of the lysosomal sulfatase that begins the breakdown of a sulfatide results in the buildup of sulfatide. As with neuronal storage diseases, a newborn with zero activity of the sulfatase may appear completely normal. Symptoms, including severe neurological and psychological retardation (and ultimately death), develop in several months as the sulfatide accumulates. The disease is called metachromatic leukodystrophy (MLD), because the stored sulfatide is metachromatic (i.e., it is negatively charged and will therefore bind certain positively charged dyes, changing their color). As mentioned in connection with gray-matter storage diseases, the fact that the stored molecule is charged may play a significant role in the pathophysiology of the disease. Sulfatide is apparently unable to cross the lysosomal membrane.

The requirement for a specific sequence of hydrolysis means that the sulfatide molecule remains intact, although only the first enzyme in the catabolic sequence is missing. Therefore, sulfatide accumulates within the lysosome. Over time, the amount of charged lipid material increases, and the material aggregates and precipitates. It eventually fills the available space in the cell, interferes with myelin's function, and produces a general breakdown of CNS function. Affected

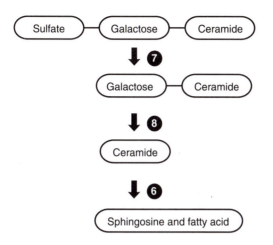

(See Table 2-1 for key to numbers representing enzymes.)

**Figure 2-6 The
Sequence of
Hydrolysis of GSLs in
White Matter**

children become increasingly retarded, since myelin is necessary for normal neuronal function.

People with different levels of residual enzyme activity may be affected at different ages of onset, but those with no active enzyme usually die before two years of age. In these situations, the disease process taking place in oligodendrocytes is analogous to GSL storage diseases in neurons.

The next enzyme in the sequence is a beta galactosidase (#8 in Table 2-1). If this enzyme is deficient, no interference with sulfatide or GM4 metabolism occurs until those molecules become cerebroside. With the hydrolysis of galactose blocked, cerebroside accumulates, but the cellular pathophysiology appears to be quite different from that of the other diseases described above. The toxic accumulation of cerebroside does not appear to occur in the oligodendrocyte (the cell in which it was made). The cerebroside may be able to leave the lysosome and the oligodendrocyte (as does the glucocerebroside in Gaucher's disease). In contrast to Gaucher's disease, however, the cerebroside appears to be taken up by microglia, the macrophages of the CNS, and significant pathology results. This disease is called Krabbe's disease, or globoid cell leukodystrophy (GLD), and is characterized by the accumulation of globoid cells. These cells, upon chemical examination, appear to be microglia with a significant, but small, buildup of cerebroside.

More importantly, the globoid cells also contain a toxic accumulation of psychosine. Psychosine, a sphingosine residue with a sugar in glycosidic linkage but no fatty acid amide, is a highly cytotoxic molecule. The accumulation of psychosine is apparently caused by a less rigorous adherence to the sequence of hydrolysis in the lysosomes of microglia, possibly related to the mesodermal origin of microglia. At any rate, the cerebroside is apparently ingested by microglia after leaving the oligodendrocytes. The microglia also lack beta galactosidase, since they have the same genome as neural cells. However, once cerebroside is present in microglial lysosomes, a small fraction of it is hydrolyzed by the next enzyme in the sequence, ceramidase (#6 in Table 2-1). This is apparently less likely to occur in oligodendrocytes, because of a more tightly controlled organization of enzymes. The removal of the fatty acid from a cerebroside creates psychosine. This probably only occurs with a small fraction of the total sphingolipid molecules. But the toxicity of psychosine is such that a severe disease results.

In one series of GLD patients in which sphingolipids were measured at autopsy, only the concentration of psychosine was roughly the same in each. Other intermediates varied widely in concentration. This fact implies that psychosine is the primary toxic molecule, and that its accumulation to a particular level results in cell death and a subsequent loss of organ function.

Deficiencies of ceramidase, the last enzyme in the sequence of degradation of a sphingolipid in white matter, have been reported, but do not seem to cause severe disability in the CNS. This may be related to the size and lack of charge of the ceramide and to the possible ability of the molecule to leave the cell of origin, as well as the CNS.

A mutation in the gene for an enzyme that has only a single copy will result in the enzyme's deficiency in all cells and tissues of the body. A ceramidase deficiency results in skin and joint pathology as well as neuropathology, produced by the accumulation of ceramides. Since significant levels of ceramides exist in the cells of the skin, where they may be part of the "waterproofing" mechanism, this enzyme deficiency results in the appearance of lipid nodules in the skin.

Storage diseases exist for the one sphingolipid in the CNS that is not a glycosphingolipid, sphingomyelin. Although it is not "characteristic" of myelin, large amounts of sphingomyelin are found in white matter. The same principles of metabolic balance apply to it as to GSLs. The only hydrolytic enzyme unique to sphingomyelin breakdown is sphingomyelinase (#9 in Table 2-1). It hydrolyzes the bond between the ceramide and the phosphoryl group, resulting in phosphoryl choline and ceramide, as shown in Figure 2-7.

A deficiency of sphingomyelinase leads to a disease called Niemann–Pick disease. The disease is commonly subdivided into types A, B, and C. Type A includes a severe neuropathy, usually resulting in death before the sixth year of life. Type B primarily affects the periphery, without significant CNS neuropathology. Type C is currently undergoing redefinition. It may not result primarily from a deficiency of sphingomyelinase and may be a distinct disease. Type C patients also have high levels of stored cholesterol, and occasionally of other lipid molecules as well. Type C is endemic in the native population of northern New

Figure 2-7 The Catabolism of Sphingomyelin

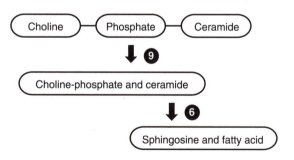

(See Table 2-1 for key to numbers representing enzymes.)

Mexico and in Quebec. It could theoretically result from mutations in a small number of individuals.

29
Self-Study Questions

SELF-STUDY QUESTIONS

Facts:

1. What are the word structures (e.g., a cerebroside is a galactose-ceramide) for gangliosides GM4, GM3, GM2, GM1, and GD1a?

2. What are the cellular sites of synthesis and catabolism of glycosphingolipids?

3. In which kind of cell is each kind of sphingolipid made and catabolized?

4. What is the sequence of lysosomal catabolism of a sulfatide? of ganglioside GM1?

5. List the products of total lysosomal digestion of a molecule of GM1 and of sulfatide.

6. What enzyme activity is missing in Tay–Sachs disease? in Gaucher's disease? in GLD? in MLD? in Niemann–Pick disease?

7. What toxic molecule accumulates in each disease referred to in question 6?

Concepts:

1. Describe the relationship between degree of enzyme deficiency and age of onset of symptoms for CNS lysosomal storage diseases.

2. Discuss the importance of autophagy in maintaining a normal, healthy CNS, and why autophagy is more important in the CNS than in other tissues.

3. Discuss the significance of an undigestible lysosomal molecule's ability to cross membranes.

BIBLIOGRAPHY

Kanfer, J.N., and Hakomori, S.I. 1983. *Sphingolipid Biochemistry*. Vol. 3 of *Handbook of Lipid Research*, edited by D. J. Hanahan. New York: Plenum Press.

Neufeld, E. 1991. Lysosomal storage diseases. *Annual Review of Biochemistry* 60: 257–280.

Scriver, C.R., Beaudet, A.L., Sly, W.S., and Valle, D. 1989. Lysosomal enzymes. In *The Metabolic Basis of Inherited Disease*, 6th ed., 1565–1839. New York: McGraw-Hill Information Services.

Synapses and Transmitters

CHAPTER 3

The Synapse

A GENERALIZED SYNAPSE

Before examining individual types of synapses, it is worthwhile to consider the manner in which synapses generally function. The synapse is the best understood means of communication between neurons, and the greatest amount of attention has been focused on this structure and its mechanisms. Some of the most fundamental concepts of brain anatomy, pharmacology, and physiology have been discovered from the study of synapses.

Chemical synapses are not the only means of communication in the CNS. There is undoubtedly a more diffuse kind of communication, produced by the release of transmitter molecules from sites other than synapses. Release of molecules from dendrites, where transmitters may make contact with other dendrites, has been known for many years. Transmitters have also recently been shown to be released in fairly large amounts from the cell body. This release into extracellular fluid may be a means of communication, or integration of communication, among neuronal groups. In addition, there are cellular contacts called "gap junctions," or "electrotonic synapses," which allow direct electrical contact and the movement of molecules other than transmitters between cells.

Among the various types of interneuronal communications, the chemical synapse allows the greatest degree of regulation or modulation. It is, therefore, thought to be the focus of integration of brain function into mental processes. There is a physiological delay in the activity of chemical synapses while transmitters diffuse from one cell to the next. This delay is usually in the range of 1 to 5 milliseconds. The postsynaptic effects caused by the transmitters last much longer. Some transmitter effects may last for seconds, and some regulatory sequelae occur over a period of hours to weeks. Both electrical and chemical events of many kinds, many of which have regulatory effects, occur at synapses. Therefore, the spatial and temporal dynamics of synapses are usually thought of as being the most important regulatory phenomena in brain function.

Anatomy

In a typical axo-dendritic synapse (Figure 3-1), there is a presynaptic axon terminal and a postsynaptic receptive region. In all cases within the brain, the

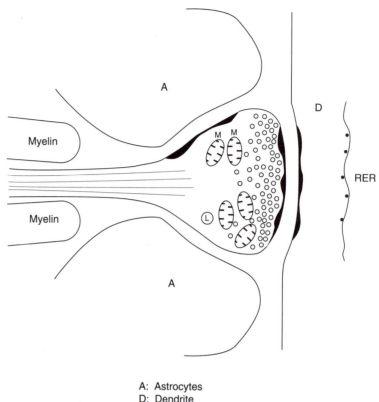

A: Astrocytes
D: Dendrite
L: Lysosome
M: Mitochondrion
RER: Rough endoplasmic reticulum

Figure 3-1 An
Axo-Dendritic Synapse

synapse is surrounded by glial cell processes, or perikarya, as well. The glial cells can be thought of as dynamic, and necessary, contributors to synaptic action. Within the presynaptic terminal are mitochondria, lysosomes, and synaptic vesicles. The synaptic vesicles, although much smaller than lysosomes, may be formed from lysosomes and may have many properties in common with them. For example, synaptic vesicles appear to have an internal pH of about 5.0, which is similar to that of lysosomes.

Over time, in any synapse, the synaptic vesicles turn over. They recycle by fusing with the plasma membrane and are then gradually returned to the terminal's cytoplasmic compartment as synaptic vesicles. This turnover probably proceeds with the help of, or through, the terminal's lysosomes.

Postsynaptic sites have been observed to have considerable membrane thickening adjacent to the membrane receptors. These areas of thickened membrane may be associated with protein synthetic machinery in the nearby cytoplasm. Such a spatial arrangement enables the postsynaptic cell to change its synthetic rate of proteins fairly quickly, in response to synaptic action.

The cytoplasm of the presynaptic terminal typically contains many of the enzymes required for synthesizing the transmitter(s) associated with that terminal. In some cases, the synthetic enzymes may be loosely associated with the cytoplasmic side of the synaptic vesicles. This arrangement allows a recently synthesized transmitter molecule to be transported and stored within the vesicle without being subject to catabolism in the cytoplasm.

Biochemistry and Physiology

An action potential, traveling down an axon to a terminal, becomes a presynaptic potential once it leaves the last myelin segment. From this point on, the presynaptic potential is propagated along the membrane incrementally, no longer by saltatory conduction. The size of the potential determines the amount of calcium mobilized along the terminal membrane. In Figure 3-2, the size of the potential refers to the area under the curve in a plot of voltage versus time. Earlier consideration of peak height alone, or the voltage difference, as the size of the potential, was shown to be inadequate, as the duration of the potential proved to be an important factor.

Calcium is necessary for all known membrane fusion events in biology. Calcium is mobilized in response to a presynaptic potential change and enters the terminal's cytoplasm, where it effects the fusion of synaptic vesicles to the plasma membrane.

Many transmitter molecules are stored in synaptic vesicles and released from them by an action potential. However, there is also evidence that not all transmitter released from synapses is from vesicles; a significant fraction may come directly from the cytoplasm. In either case, transmitter molecules are released from the presynaptic cell and enter the synaptic cleft. Once in the cleft, it is necessary for the

Figure 3-2 Presynaptic Potentials

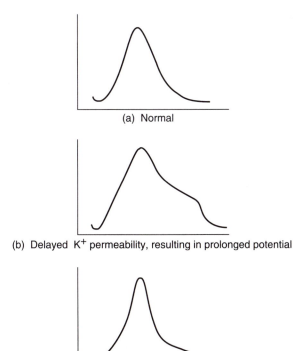

(a) Normal

(b) Delayed K^+ permeability, resulting in prolonged potential

(c) Enhanced K^+ permeability, resulting in shortened potential

transmitter molecules to diffuse across the extracellular space to the postsynaptic membrane, before interaction with that cell's receptors is possible.

Within the cleft, there is a large amount of proteoglycan (a complex **glycoprotein** material that is highly negatively charged). This glycoprotein in the synaptic cleft has enough structural integrity itself and provides enough structure to the cleft to hold both the presynaptic and the postsynaptic membranes together, even after the cells have been disrupted (by homogenization, for example). It is possible to prepare particles from brain, called synaptosomes, which consist of the entire presynaptic terminal, broken off and resealed below the last myelin segment. Such synaptosomes also contain the proteoglycan from the synaptic cleft and the patch of postsynaptic membrane with its receptors.

Within the synaptic vesicles, the neurotransmitter(s) characteristic of the presynaptic cell are stored with other molecules. In order to pack a large number of transmitter molecules into a vesicle, it is necessary to deal with the osmotic problem. That is, a large number of molecules packed into a small volume will cause water to flow into that volume, in order to equalize the concentrations of particles on each side of the membrane. Without some kind of protection of the synaptic vesicles, this inward flow of water might cause the vesicles to burst.

In some synapses there is a "storage" protein known to exist within the vesicle. Each storage molecule, a glycosaminoglycan (complex glycoprotein), binds a large number of transmitter molecules to it. This in effect reduces the large number of particles to one, thereby reducing the osmotic pressure within the vesicle. Most transmitter molecules have positive charges, and thereby can bind electrostatically to the negative charges on the carbohydrate residues of the storage molecule. More specific kinds of binding may also occur.

More than one kind of transmitter may be present in a single terminal and in a single vesicle. Depending on the kind of neuron, it is not uncommon to find both a biogenic amine and a **peptide** transmitter in the same terminal. For example, acetylcholine (Chapter 5) is often found with vasoactive intestinal peptide (VIP) (Chapter 8), and dopamine (Chapter 6) is often found with cholecystokinin (CCK-8) (Chapter 8).

In addition to transmitters and storage proteins, synaptic vesicles contain metal ions (e.g., magnesium), ATP, cofactors, and a few enzymes, depending on the cell. One or more of the enzymes involved in the synthesis of some transmitters (e.g., noradrenaline and adrenaline) may also be contained in the vesicle. These are usually enzymes that are employed later in the synthetic sequence. All of these molecules are released, or at least given access to the cleft, after the vesicle has fused with the cell's plasma membrane. A fraction of these ancillary molecules then are carried out of the CNS into the bloodstream via the flow of extracellular fluid. The amount of this release is in direct proportion to the general level of activity of that transmitter's synapses. It is therefore possible, at least theoretically, to measure substances in the blood that correlate with specific CNS transmitter function.

After the transmitters are released into the cleft, the first receptors they encounter are those on the extracellular surface of the cell that released them. These autoreceptors are usually inhibitory, meaning that they inhibit further release of the transmitter from the same cell as long as the concentration of the transmitter is high in the extracellular fluid space adjacent to the presynaptic membrane. Autoreceptors also are often structurally and functionally distinct from the receptors on the postsynaptic membrane in the same synapse.

In addition to the transmitter and its accompanying enzymes and storage proteins, ATP is released into the cleft from the vesicles. This extracellular ATP is apparently quickly degraded by phosphatases, becoming successively ADP and AMP.

On the plasma membrane of the glial cells, facing the extracellular compartment, is a 5′ nucleotidase. This enzyme is attached to the membrane by a glycosidic "tail," which is anchored to the glial membrane by a phosphoinositol residue. This physical arrangement allows the 5′ **nucleotidase** to "sweep" a volume of extracellular fluid. In doing so, it hydrolyzes the remaining 5′ phosphate from AMP, converting it to adenosine. Adenosine is known to be an active molecule in brain, being variously thought of as a transmitter at its own synapses or as a modulator of other synapses. The production of adenosine by the mechanism just described may be a general means for increasing blood flow to a functioning synapse. If ATP is present in all or most synaptic vesicles, regardless of the transmitters stored with it, its presence in the cleft, and the subsequent formation of adenosine, could be a universal signal. Adenosine is able to activate **adenylyl cyclase,** which is associated with vasodilation and increased cerebral blood flow.

After diffusing across the cleft, transmitter molecules are able to bind to postsynaptic receptors and to effect whatever cellular changes are specific for those receptors in the postsynaptic cells. The two major types of effects are either excitatory (producing excitatory postsynaptic potentials, or epsp's) or inhibitory (producing inhibitory postsynaptic potentials, ipsp's). Excitatory potentials depolarize the postsynaptic cell, reducing the negative charge inside the cell relative to the outside. Inhibitory potentials, for the most part, are those that increase the negative charge inside cells in relation to the outside. This inhibitory effect is a **hyperpolarization.** Postsynaptic responses that inhibit the hyperpolarization of the cell are considered epsp's, and those that block excitation are considered ipsp's.

Each of these kinds of postsynaptic potentials can be produced by various molecular mechanisms, some of which will be discussed later (Chapters 10 and 11). An excitatory, depolarizing response results in an increased likelihood of the postsynaptic cell's reaching its threshold for firing. That is, the postsynaptic cell is more likely to form an action potential of its own. Ipsp's, also produced by a variety of mechanisms, make it more difficult for the postsynaptic cell to fire an action potential.

Although it is not entirely clear at present what molecular signals are used, it is clear that postsynaptic cells communicate with their associated presynaptic terminals. If the postsynaptic cell is firing at a rate that is either significantly greater than usual or significantly less than usual, this change is signalled to the presynaptic terminal. Depending on the particular synapse and the transmitters involved, this change of postsynaptic cell activity may result in a change in activity of the presynaptic cell in the direction of **homeostasis,** or compensation. The molecules most frequently implicated as having this messenger function are lipids, produced from portions of the membrane phospholipids around the synapse. For example, there is evidence that **arachidonic acid,** previously regarded only as a precursor for **prostaglandins** and other **eicosanoids,** may be one such signal. Some of the prostaglandins (i.e., signal molecules made from arachidonic acid) have also been suspected of having this role.

In one synaptic event, transmitters are released, diffuse across the cleft, and produce a characteristic postsynaptic effect. There must also be a mechanism to terminate the transmitter's activity. The two basic mechanisms for inactivation of transmitters in a synaptic cleft are catabolism (within the cleft) and removal of the transmitter from the cleft by uptake into a nearby cell. Acetylcholine is known to be hydrolyzed in the cleft, which ends its action. Neuropeptides also appear to be hydrolyzed extracellularly, although all the details of this process are not clear. Hydrolysis destroys the transmitter molecule, which must then be resynthesized. New synthesis requires an input of energy, as well as a fresh supply of some substrates.

Most other known neurotransmitters appear to be recycled, starting with a re-uptake mechanism. Re-uptake into the axon terminal from which the transmitter was released allows the molecules to be stored in vesicles and reused without a significant energy or substrate requirement. In at least one case, however (gamma amino butyric acid), the uptake from the synaptic cleft is into the nearby glial cells. In these astrocytes, the transmitter is further metabolized and a precursor molecule is returned to the axon terminal. The uptake is by Na^+-coupled **symport,** which is the most common mechanism for moving amino acids, simple sugars, and neurotransmitters across membranes. In this process, the **symporter** is an integral membrane molecule, in the plasma membrane of the presynaptic terminal. It will transport the neurotransmitter across the membrane only if there is a Na^+ bound to it at the same time. Both the sodium ion and the transmitter molecule are transported into the cytoplasm. The energy necessary for this transport is therefore provided by the Na^+ gradient across the plasma membrane. Most commonly, Na^+ is present at about 100 mM in extracellular fluid and only about 10 mM in the cytoplasm. This tenfold gradient will drive a transport of transmitter across the membrane, even if the transmitter's concentration is higher in the cytoplasm than in the cleft.

Despite the existence of re-uptake mechanisms, however, all neurotransmitters must undergo catabolism eventually. In most cases in which transmitters undergo re-uptake into their presynaptic terminals, their catabolism is intracellular. Therefore, within any particular axon terminal there are several simultaneous and competing processes involving the existing pool of transmitter molecules. The transmitter molecules recently removed from the cleft may be combined with those just synthesized in the cytoplasm. This pool is then subject to release into the cleft from the cytoplasm, storage in synaptic vesicles, or catabolism by intracellular enzymes. Quantitative estimates of transmitters known to undergo re-uptake and/or catabolism in this manner indicate that about 60 percent of the pool released into the cleft is stored in vesicles and subsequently rereleased. A minority of the transmitter is catabolized, as much as 40 percent; the percentage is relatively constant for each synaptic event. Therefore, the total amount of a transmitter that is catabolized each day, even of those that are predominantly recycled, is proportional to the number of times that transmitter's synapses have been fired. A few transmitters, mostly biogenic amines (see below), are catabolized to characteristic end products within the CNS. The levels of these end products can be determined in **cerebrospinal fluid** (CSF), as a measure of the total activity of that transmitter in the person's recent past. This technique has been used to study the involvement of particular neurotransmitters in psychiatric diseases, and will be discussed in more detail later.

In an overview of the synapses of the mammalian brain, it is useful to categorize neurotransmitters into three general classes. These classes do not have sharp boundaries, but the distinctions are useful when considering the types of physiological functions in which each neurotransmitter is involved and its synaptic dynamics. The classes vary according to the types of molecules, their concentration in whole brain, the locations of their associated axon terminals and receptors, the kinds of receptors, and the duration of their receptor effects.

Global Neurotransmitters

The first class, the global neurotransmitters, composed of amino acids, is found in largest concentration in whole brain and has the widest distribution throughout the brain. Most neurons are responsive to amino acids, and many may be subjected to them continuously. Amino acid transmitters can be thought of as setting the overall excitation/inhibition "tone" of the CNS. Large changes in the overall ratio of excitatory to inhibitory amino acid transmitters are associated with global changes in brain function. Increased excitatory amino acids are associated with generalized excitation or seizures. Increasing inhibitory amino acids may lead to generalized depression or even stupor or coma.

Functionally Specific Neurotransmitters

The second class, the functionally specific neurotransmitters, is predominantly composed of biogenic amines and some of the **peptides.** These transmitters are found in more restricted locations and are often associated with specific groups of neurons, called nuclei. These transmitters, although present in high concentrations within the neurons that synthesize them and in immediately surrounding areas, are not generally found in large concentration throughout the brain. They are also more functionally specific than amino acid transmitters. Many of them can be associated with more or less specific physiological functions of the organism. For example, increasing the release of serotonin in specific locations can produce particular changes in sleep patterns and sexual activity. Increasing the release of certain peptides causes changes in the organism's experience of hunger or thirst.

Modulatory Neurotransmitters

The third class of transmitters, the modulatory neurotransmitters, are all peptides and are generally found in low concentration. They are not associated with the activation or cessation of specific physiological functions, but rather with their modification. That is, they function as "modulators," often of the activity of second-level transmitters. Many such neuropeptides are released at presynaptic synapses—meaning that they are released onto the presynaptic terminal of another synapse, as shown in Figure 3-3. Presynaptic inhibition or potentiation, as determined by the transmitters and receptors involved, is restricted to diminution or augmentation of the action of the primary synapse. This primary synapse often uses a different transmitter. Therefore, the effects of modulatory transmitters are

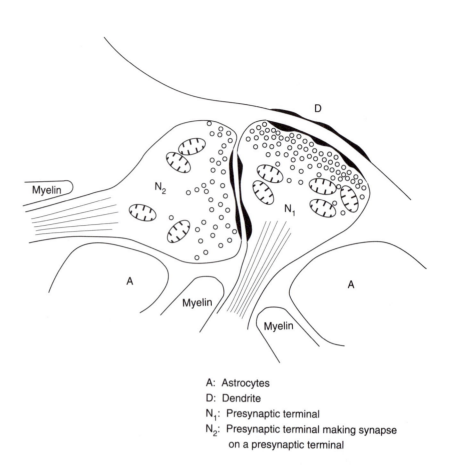

A: Astrocytes
D: Dendrite
N_1: Presynaptic terminal
N_2: Presynaptic terminal making synapse
    on a presynaptic terminal

**Figure 3-3 A Presynaptic
Synapse**

quantitative in nature (i.e., modulatory) and are usually not associated qualitatively with specific physiology.

These transmitters often have strong binding constants for their receptors. The binding constants (K_D) for enkephalins, for example, are on the order of 10^{-10} M. Such tight binding is necessary for the molecule to produce an effect, as the transmitter may not be present, even in its own synaptic clefts, in high concentration.

Partly as a result of this tight binding, these peptides also typically have longer-lasting postsynaptic effects than other transmitters. Some peptide-induced cellular effects last for seconds. Some peptides, e.g., bradykinin, produce multiple effects, presumably at multiple receptor sites. These effects can even be opposite in nature. That is, a single pulse of synaptic peptide release can result in an initial depolarization, followed after a few hundred milliseconds by a hyperpolarization.

SYNAPTIC REGULATORY MECHANISMS

The regulation of synaptic function is quite complex, with regulatory mechanisms occurring in different time frames, on different kinds of molecules, and in different compartments. **Allosteric** regulatory changes, which are modifications of the structure of protein molecules, typically occur in microseconds, whereas changes in receptor concentrations require many minutes, or even hours or days. Changes in levels of synthesis of regulatory proteins, which may involve different levels of gene expression, may take weeks or even longer to appear. Clinical syndromes that may involve long-term changes in receptor levels, among other things, may take years to develop. There are also many levels of synaptic regulatory mechanisms between these two extremes.

The different time periods for different regulatory phenomena are confusing enough, but there are also regulatory mechanisms that modify function in opposite directions and thereby counteract each other. Biologists have long been familiar with the concept of homeostatic regulation, whereby a system responds to a change by adapting to it, incorporating the change into the system in such a way that it no longer causes the same effect. This kind of regulation, called **negative feedback (NFB),** is thought to be most important or most common.

Homeostatic, or NFB, regulatory changes of synaptic function can lead in the long term to an internal compensation for the acute effect of a drug. This is especially likely when there is chronic repetition of the short-term effect. For example, the addition of an inhibitory drug to an excitatory synapse produces inhibition, by definition. If the drug is administered over the long term (i.e., chronically), there will be a compensatory long-term regulatory change in synaptic activity. The compensation is increased excitatory activity, making it more difficult for the drug to produce an inhibition. Therefore, the synapse works at approximately the normal rate in the presence of the drug, but it will work at a higher level than normal in the absence of the drug. Thus, the baseline level of synaptic function moves back toward the original in the presence of the drug. This kind of overall change is seen in the development of **tolerance** and addiction to many drugs.

Homeostasis has been called the "wisdom of the body" and was long thought to be the only kind of regulation. Examples of homeostatic regulation in synapses are the well-known phenomena of "down regulation" and "up regulation." In both cases, a relatively long-term change in the activity of a synapse results in a compensatory change in receptor number. If the bundle of axons innervating a muscle fiber is cut, the long-term lack of stimulation to the fiber results in its increasing the number of receptors and the area of distribution of receptors on the fiber. This is up regulation. Once up regulation occurs, small amounts of transmitter, much less than those necessary to cause a measurable response before the cut, will produce an enhanced response.

Down regulation is the opposite phenomenon. The number of receptor molecules is decreased in response to an increased (relatively long-term) activation of the synapse, such as an increased release of transmitter. This effect, also in response to multiple stimulations, results in the overall activity of the synapses being restored toward its original level. Another important point illustrated by these phenomena is that the postsynaptic response to a transmitter is not simply a function of the amount of transmitter released. It is determined by the product of the concentrations of both transmitter and receptor. Therefore, increased synaptic activity can be achieved by increasing either factor.

Changes can also occur in the opposite direction, under certain circumstances and in some synapses. These kinds of regulatory modifications are called

positive feed forward (PFF). They are important in learning, for example. In PFF, long-term regulatory changes occur in the same direction as the short-term effect. Once having activated a pathway involved in walking, for example, it becomes easier to activate that pathway again. The converse, inhibiting a pathway, is that it becomes easier to inhibit the same activity in the future, after it has been inhibited in the short term. Obviously, the study of these (higher) regulatory mechanisms, which determine whether NFB or PFF kinds of effects will occur in response to a particular synaptic change, is of major importance in understanding the mechanisms of brain function. It is also an extraordinarily complex study.

The CNS of higher mammals has a large capacity for the positive feed forward (PFF) kind of regulation. (One can call these changes **homotropic,** to distinguish them from homeostatic.) This kind of regulation is essential for higher, cognitive learning, and may operate in a way that is physiologically similar to the regulation of **motor** learning, as in the example cited above. It is clear that if homeostasis were perfectly effective, cognitive learning would be impossible. However, all higher mammals have the ability to incorporate changes into the nervous system in response to environmental stimuli (see Chapter 12).

SELF-STUDY QUESTIONS

Facts:

1. What types of molecules are found in the synaptic vesicles of a particular synapse?

2. In what parts of the cell do the different steps of transmitter metabolism occur?

Concepts:

1. Describe the role of Ca^{++} in exocytosis.

2. Describe the type of synaptic inactivation (i.e., either hydrolysis or uptake) for each kind of transmitter.

3. Describe the mechanism of Na^+ coupled symport.

4. Discuss the differences in function between postsynaptic and presynaptic receptors for the same transmitter.

5. Describe the three general classes of neurotransmitter and the characteristics of each class in terms of total amount of transmitter, associations with brain functions, duration of effect, and types of receptors.

6. Describe the use of transmitter catabolites for the study of disease.

7. Describe the production and effects of adenosine in synapses.

8. Describe at least five macromolecules specialized for binding the transmitter in a single synapse.

9. Describe the two different directions for regulatory changes in receptor concentration.

BIBLIOGRAPHY

Augustine, G.J., Charlton, M.P., and Smith, S.J. 1987. Calcium action in synaptic transmitter release. *Annual Review of Neuroscience* 10: 633–693.

Erulkar, S.D. 1989. Chemically mediated synaptic transmission: An overview. In *Basic Neurochemistry*, edited by G. Siegel, B. Agranoff, R.W. Albers, and P. Molinoff. New York: Raven Press.

Trimble, W.S., Linial, M., and Scheller, R.H. 1991. Cellular and molecular biology of the presynaptic nerve terminal. *Annual Review of Neuroscience* 14: 93–122.

CHAPTER 4

Amino Acid Neurotransmitters

GENERAL PRINCIPLES

Amino acids are found throughout the CNS in higher concentration than in any other tissue of the body. The liver regulates blood amino acid concentration by using "excess" amino acids for urea synthesis. Whenever the concentration of amino acids in the blood is elevated above the normal level of about 3 to 4.5 mM, an increase in urea synthesis results. In contrast, brain maintains a combined total of free amino acids of about 30 mM. Free amino acids in both brain and liver are required to support high rates of protein synthesis. The brain does not use amino acids for **gluconeogenesis** or for the synthesis of urea to any significant degree; rather, brain has many specialized uses for amino acids in connection with both metabolic regulation and neurotransmission.

The response of most CNS neurons to amino acid neurotransmitters is either inhibition or excitation. This implies that most neurons contain specific receptors for those amino acids that are neurotransmitters. Most neurons likely receive a large amino acid neurotransmitter input in vivo. This is supported by in vivo observations described below. The amino acids, or their derivatives, that are present in highest quantity in the CNS are glutamate, aspartate, N-acetyl aspartate, gamma amino butyric acid, and glycine. Taurine, serine, proline, and alanine are also present in significant concentrations. There is some evidence that each of these free amino acids may play a role in neurotransmission. In addition to free amino acids, the brain contains a significant concentration of **dipeptides** and dipeptide derivatives that may play functional roles in neurotransmission. The most prominent dipeptide is N-acetyl-asp-glu. All the above amino acids and derivatives can produce, in particular circumstances, a postsynaptic effect when applied to the plasma membrane of neurons. Figure 4-1 shows the structures of the five most common CNS amino acids in their predominant ionization states at neutral pH.

All known amino acid neurotransmitters, as well as those that are likely candidates, are **non-essential** amino acids—that is, animal tissues can synthesize them in situ. These synthetic pathways use, for the most part, the same enzymes used by the liver, although their regulation may be specific to brain. For example, the synthetic pathway for glycine branches from glycolysis at 3-phospho-glyceric acid. This pathway may include a unique, regulatory isozyme in brain.

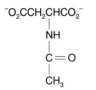

N-acetyl aspartate

$^-O_2CCH_2CH_2CH(NH_3^+)CO_2^-$

Glutamate

$^-O_2CCH_2CH(NH_3^+)CO_2^-$

Aspartate

$^+H_3NCH_2CH_2CH_2CO_2^-$

Gamma-amino butyrate (GABA)

$^+H_3NCH_2CO_2^-$

Glycine

Figure 4-1 The Predominant Amino Acids in Brain

The fact that only non-essential amino acids are used as neurotransmitters emphasizes a significant point regarding the ability of amino acids to cross the blood–brain barrier. Molecules known to function as neurotransmitters do not have a direct, net transport into brain from the periphery, or vice versa. Neurotransmitters such as noradrenaline, serotonin, and dopamine are prevented from equilibrating across the blood–brain barrier by virtue of both their positive charge and the presence of catabolic enzymes in the endothelial cells of the cerebral vasculature. Peptide transmitters and modulators are also charged, and are subject to rapid enzymatic degradation. Such a system is desirable from an evolutionary point of view, in that these molecules can have functionally distinct roles in brain and in other tissues. For example, serotonin and noradrenaline have roles in maintaining blood pressure that are functionally separate from their roles as neurotransmitters (in the CNS).

The amino acid neurotransmitters similarly do not equilibrate between the brain and the bloodstream. Glutamate, aspartate, glycine, and GABA do not have a net transport across the blood–brain barrier and do not equilibrate across this barrier. As a general rule, the blood–brain barrier excludes transport of non-essential amino acids, whereas **essential** amino acids have more or less specific transporters that allow a net uptake. Since essential amino acids are needed for protein synthesis and no human cell can synthesize them, there must be specific mechanisms to supply adequate amounts of them to neural cells. A major exception to this generalization appears to occur in the hypothalamus, much of which does not exhibit an effective blood–brain barrier.

EXCITATORY AMINO ACIDS

Glutamate and aspartate (or N-acetyl aspartate) are thought of as the major excitatory amino acid transmitters. As a generalization, dicarboxylic amino acids (i.e., those with two negatively charged carboxyl groups) tend to be excitatory transmitters. This may be true even if their amino groups are protected by acetylation (see Figure 4-1). Glutamate is more widespread in the CNS than aspartate. Most neurons have glutamate receptors and are activated by its contact. Aspartate and its derivatives, although they occur widely in lower concentrations, are most highly concentrated in the motor (ventral) spinal cord. Aspartate appears to be the major excitatory amino acid in this area, controlling many muscle movements.

Synaptic function has traditionally been conceptualized in terms of the transmitter molecule. Such an emphasis led to some oversimplifications, i.e., particular transmitters were judged to have only a single brain function. Current research has led to a greater emphasis on the role of receptors. Transmitters are known to have various, and sometimes conflicting, cellular effects, each resulting from the activation of different receptors. One particular kind of receptor, therefore, is more likely to be associated with a particular function than its transmitter is. The specific function is also dependent on the specific cellular location of the receptor within the brain, however.

One result of increased focus on receptor function (as opposed to transmitter function) is an emphasis on receptor specificity. If, for example, a receptor is excitatory, the cell containing the receptor is stimulated by its activation, regardless of the **ligand.** For example, excitatory amino acid receptors, often referred to as "glutamate" receptors, may be activated by other naturally occurring amino acids or derivatives of amino acids, such as aspartate or N-acetyl aspartate. This process, whereby a single receptor is able to respond to more than one ligand, is somewhat analogous to the genetic code, in which a single amino acid may be specified by more than one codon. This concept, that different molecules can produce the same result, is called degeneracy. In this case, different transmitter molecules, or even metabolic products of transmitters, can activate the same receptor, thereby producing the same effect in the postsynaptic cell. The receptor, not necessarily the transmitter, is associated with a particular cellular response.

Glutamate (i.e., excitatory amino acid) receptors are now often divided into five classes: AMPA, K, NMDA, LAP4, and ACPD. The initials stand for drugs that activate each receptor selectively. Since glutamate itself can stimulate all five, the different receptors can be distinguished from each other only by selective drug binding (see Chapter 9 for a more extensive discussion of this phenomenon).

Ion channels are opened by an allosteric effect in response to the binding of an acceptable transmitter. Allosterism refers to a kind of regulatory process that many protein molecules can undergo. In allosterism, a conformational change in a protein is induced by the binding of an appropriate ligand to the allosteric site on the molecule, and this conformational change affects the protein's activity. Enzymes were first discovered to be allosteric, but it is now known that many important regulatory proteins, from receptors to gene regulators, operate in this way. Allosteric regulation is a fundamental biochemical process.

Allosteric binding is different from substrate binding (as in the case of an enzyme) in at least two ways. The allosteric binding site is some distance away from the substrate site on the molecule, and the allosteric ligand is not changed by the protein. On the contrary, the binding of the allosteric ligand to the protein results in a change in the structure of the protein, which further changes its activity. For this reason, it is more common to refer to allosteric binding constants as K_D

and substrate binding constants as **Km.** For example, the allosteric binding of ATP to the glycolytic enzyme phosphofructokinase (PFK) raises the Km of PFK for its substrate. The enzyme is thereby inhibited, and the ATP molecule is unchanged.

Allosteric enzymes are composed of more than one subunit, as there must be binding sites of different kinds in different places on the molecule. Neurotransmitter receptors are also composed of several subunits. The transmitter binds to the receptor complex, resulting in a change in the protein's structure, and the transmitter is not itself changed by this interaction. In the case of the excitatory amino acid K and AMPA receptors, the allosteric changes in their structures allow an **ionophore** to form in the cell's membrane, which then allows a change in relative concentration of sodium and potassium ions across the membrane. Water and other substances also pass through the channel, of course. A large number of receptors are now known to function in this way, as allosteric protein complexes that respond to their appropriate ligands by forming membrane channels. K and AMPA are but two of several types of receptors that will be discussed in more detail in Chapter 9.

LAP4, ACPD, and NMDA receptors are significantly different in their mechanisms from the first two, although they are also allosteric. These receptors also cause activation of the cell, but they do so by increasing the cytoplasmic concentration of calcium ion. NMDA receptors allow the entry of Ca^{++} from extracellular sources, whereas activation of LAP4 and ACPD receptors results in the release of Ca^{++} from endoplasmic reticulum into cytoplasm.

The regulation of NMDA receptors is complex, involving several different allosteric ligands and also depending on the level of depolarization of the cell. Such a complex regulatory system, involving both chemical factors and a cellular factor (the voltage across the membrane), assures that NMDA receptors are activated only under precisely controlled conditions (see Chapter 9). This is necessary because NMDA receptors can activate the cells that contain them to dangerously high levels.

NMDA receptors are thought to be involved in many kinds of desirable long-term alterations of cellular functioning. Such long-term changes in cells can also determine long-term changes in the synaptic networks that include these cells. For example, NMDA receptors may play an important role in learning (Chapter 12), converting temporarily activated synaptic networks into relatively permanent memories. They also may be involved in the development of epileptic foci, a process that has some similarity to learning. Finally, the ability to depolarize cells to this extent may, if imperfectly controlled, result in neuronal death. Cell death may occur as a result of overstimulation of the cell's catabolic pathways to the point of self-digestion. Each of these physiological processes is now a major focus of research.

INHIBITORY AMINO ACIDS

Glycine and gamma amino butyric acid (GABA) are the two inhibitory amino acid transmitters found in highest concentration in the CNS. Their patterns of localization are somewhat analogous to those of aspartate and glutamate, respectively. Glycine is distributed less generally throughout the CNS than GABA and is partially localized to neurons in the ventral spinal cord, as is aspartate. GABA is concentrated in the dorsal spinal cord, as is glutamate. Both glutamate and GABA are also found in high concentration throughout the brain itself. It may be reasonable to think of these pairs as endogenous excitatory/inhibitory pairs of transmitters, particularly at the level of the spinal cord.

GABA and glutamate are also similar in that most cerebral cells respond to them, providing evidence for the general occurrence of both GABA and glutamate receptors. This pairing constitutes a generalized excitatory/inhibitory system. One characteristic of this first level of neurotransmitter function is that the overall ratio of excitatory and inhibitory amino acid activity may set the basic activation/inhibition "tone" of the CNS.

The most common postsynaptic receptors for both GABA and glycine are inhibitory Cl^- channels. In each case, the allosteric binding of molecules of the transmitter opens the receptor's channel. This allows Cl^- ions to move toward equilibrium across the plasma membrane. Regardless of the direction of net movement of Cl^- ions, the membrane then moves toward stabilization as a "chloride membrane" (i.e., a membrane at the equilibrium potential for chloride ion) and, as such, becomes more resistant to depolarization. Cl^- receptors are therefore inhibitory.

The main postsynaptic GABA and glycine receptors are similar, which illustrates a developing theme in receptor structure. As more receptors are cloned, it has become apparent that they sort out into a few families, although each family has a surprisingly large number of members. Each family has common structural features, including the number and kind of membrane-spanning sequences and the number and location of transmitter-binding sites and other regulatory sites. There is reason to believe that evolution has been highly conservative, keeping design motifs and using them frequently. There is also great heterogeneity, as the number of specific protein sequences that bind to any particular transmitter is much greater than most investigators would have predicted. It is likely that many different receptor structures have evolved from the same original ion channel, as is clearly possible in the case of the inhibitory amino acids.

The most well-known glycine receptor is also the primary site of action of strychnine. Strychnine is a competitive inhibitor of glycine's binding. Since glycine is inhibitory, strychnine is therefore excitatory. This is a simple example of **disinhibition** (i.e., producing excitation by inhibiting an inhibitory action), which is common in the CNS. It is observed in the action of exogenous drugs (for example, strychnine) and in endogenous mechanisms at the molecular, cellular, and multi-cellular levels.

GABA has at least two different, well-characterized receptors: the $GABA_A$ receptor, mentioned above, which has been cloned and thoroughly studied for many years, and the $GABA_B$ receptor. The $GABA_A$ receptor is a Cl^- ion channel and is also one site of action of many commonly used drugs, such as alcohol, benzodiazepines, and barbiturates. Both alcohol and the benzodiazepines have a stimulatory effect on the $GABA_A$ receptor, and are therefore inhibitory drugs. They work not as direct activators of the receptor but by allosterically enhancing the effects of GABA—that is, they have an allosteric effect on an allosteric **effector.** This may be an important part of the mechanism by which each of these drugs produces the psychological effects desired by the user.

METABOLISM OF AMINO ACID NEUROTRANSMITTERS

Amino acid transmitters, as a result of their status as non-essential amino acids, can be synthesized by the normal complement of enzymes that the brain shares with other tissues (such as liver). The major amino acid transmitters are synthesized from glycolytic and **citric acid cycle** intermediates. The CNS contains some enzymes that are specific to it, either in that the enzyme does not exist in other tissues or in that the CNS contains a special isozyme. For example, peripheral tissues do not use significant quantities of GABA, and both the major synthetic enzymes (glutamic acid decarboxylase, or GAD) and catabolic enzymes (GABA transaminase, or GABA-T) of GABA metabolism are, therefore, highly concentrated in brain. Evolution may have utilized this peculiarity to devise a system of metabolic protection of the brain in cases of **hypoglycemia** or **hypoxia.** It is theorized that the protective mechanism is dependent on the ratio of glutamate to GABA. This ratio, in any particular region of the brain or in any particular synaptic region, sets the level of excitation/inhibition. Although the specifics of this hypothesis have not been shown, evidence from both experimental systems and clinical observations support this concept.

Figure 4-2 shows the metabolism of GABA. The hypothesis mentioned above centers on GABA, since its metabolism uses enzymes that are relatively unique to the CNS. The flow of carbon atoms into GABA from citric acid cycle intermediates and the return of the four carbons of GABA back into the citric acid cycle is often called the "GABA shunt." The net effect of the GABA shunt on energy metabolism is to bypass the citric acid cycle's production of one NADH from the decarboxylation of alpha-keto glutarate and of one GTP from the hydrolysis of succinyl CoA.

THE METABOLIC RESPONSE TO HYPOXIA AND HYPOGLYCEMIA

One of the products of the GABA-T reaction is succinic semialdehyde (Figure 4-2). It is quickly removed from the reaction site by oxidation to succinate. Prompt removal of aldehydes is necessary because of their reactivity (i.e., their toxicity). Prompt removal of one product means that the GABA-T reaction, unlike

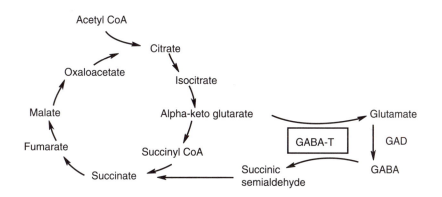

Figure 4-2 The Relationship Between the Citric Acid Cycle and the GABA Shunt

other aminotransferases (or transaminases), usually proceeds in one direction only. Other aminotransferases work equally well in either direction.

In addition, GABA-T is specialized to the exclusive use of alpha-keto glutarate as the acceptor of GABA's amino group. This substrate specificity is greater than that of other aminotransferases, so GABA-T is unusual in two ways. These characteristics of GABA-T result in GABA's catabolism being sensitive to the activity of the citric acid cycle, as explained below.

Aminotransferases are not allosteric enzymes and, therefore, are usually at metabolic equilibrium. As is true of all equilibria reactions, they are normally controlled only by mass action. If the concentration of either product or substrate is increased, the reaction will proceed in the other direction, in order to reach equilibrium again. Therefore, the reaction rate of GABA-T, an aminotransferase that is both unidirectional and highly specific for one of its substrates, is determined by the concentrations of its two substrates (Figure 4-2).

Glutamate is a part of the GABA system, since one molecule of glutamate is produced for each molecule of GABA that is transaminated. Glutamate is both a major excitatory transmitter and the immediate precursor of GABA, which is the major inhibitory transmitter. This metabolic design produces an interesting interaction of amino acids and CNS function.

The two substrates of GABA-T are GABA, the predominant inhibitory neurotransmitter, and alpha-keto glutarate, the product of a rate-controlling enzyme of the citric acid cycle. Whenever the citric acid cycle is inhibited, the concentration of alpha-keto glutarate falls. The reaction rate of GABA-T will also fall as a result. No other catabolic mechanism for GABA is available, and its concentration will therefore rise. This system leads to a decrease in the cell's glutamate/GABA ratio. A generalized lowering of this ratio may lead to a lowering of the tonic level of activity of all amino-acid-sensitive neurons.

If such a metabolic mechanism exists, one of its consequences is an inhibition of brain electrical activity in response to an inhibition of brain mitochondrial metabolism. For example, in hypoxia (or carbon monoxide or cyanide poisoning, which produce similar effects), this mechanism would elevate GABA, possibly resulting in a generalized inhibition. A decrease in the overall level of synaptic activity reduces the brain's ATP use by Na^+, K^+, ATPase. The response of this system to an inhibition of citric acid cycle metabolism may help prevent the cell's **energy charge** from becoming so low that an auto-destructive process is initiated (see Chapter 14). One evolutionary advantage of the GABA shunt may be such an ability to delay metabolic "exhaustion" and its potentially destructive consequences. This mechanism would be advantageous in any condition in which the energy charge in the cell's cytoplasm was low at the same time the citric acid cycle was inhibited, which could result in cell damage. Such a condition can arise with a deficiency of either of the brain's two obligatory substrates, glucose and oxygen.

The large majority of oxygen used by the brain is used by cytochrome oxidase, the final enzyme in the electron transport system. When the oxygen supply becomes too low to sustain this enzyme's reaction, the entire electron transport system is inhibited. The electron transport system, although quite complex in structure, is entirely contained within the mitochondrial inner membrane. The entire membrane functions somewhat like an enzyme whose substrates are NADH (generated within the mitochondrion) and oxygen. Therefore, when O_2 is deficient, the concentration of NADH rises. NADH is the major allosteric inhibitor of isocitrate dehydrogenase, which is the primary regulatory enzyme for the citric acid cycle. Inhibition reduces this enzyme's production of alpha-keto glutarate, therefore causing GABA's concentration to rise, in turn, by the above mechanisms.

When glucose is low, the result is a decreased glycolytic production of pyruvate. When pyruvate in the mitochondrion is lowered, less acetyl **coenzyme** A can be made from it. The citric acid cycle is also regulated, in part, by the concentrations of acetyl CoA and oxaloacetate, as they can be rate-limiting substrates for the enzyme that synthesizes citric acid. Therefore, hypoglycemia also inhibits the citric acid cycle while energy charge is low elsewhere in the cell.

THE METABOLIC RESPONSE TO VITAMIN B$_6$ DEFICIENCY

The two enzymes most specific for the CNS in the GABA shunt are GAD and GABA-T. Both enzymes require pyridoxal phosphate (PLP) as a **catalytic cofactor.** PLP is synthesized by the cell from the vitamin pyroxidine, or vitamin B$_6$. GABA-T, however, differs from GAD in that it binds the cofactor in covalent linkage (by a **Schiff base**) and the decarboxylase does not. Therefore, the decarboxylase is dependent upon binding PLP from the available soluble pool of the coenzyme, and has a measurable Km for this interaction. This difference in the two enzymes' interaction with PLP is a possible explanation for the only known symptom of vitamin B$_6$ deficiency, an increased susceptibility to seizures. This might be explained by the mechanism described below.

When the dietary intake of vitamin B$_6$, or pyridoxine, is such that the body cannot maintain adequate levels of PLP, the synthesis of GABA is primarily affected. Decreased levels of PLP inhibit GAD activity more than GABA-T, because the covalent linkage with the latter enzyme prevents the loss of the cofactor. In this case, production of GABA falls in relation to its catabolism, resulting in an *increase* in the glutamate/GABA ratio. This situation is, therefore, expected to increase the irritability of the CNS, producing a greater likelihood of seizures. This effect is in the opposite direction from that induced by hypoxia. Interestingly, an overdose of vitamin B$_6$ may produce the same effect as a deficiency. The vitamin form of the coenzyme, pyridoxine, has some similarity of structure to pyridoxal phosphate, lacking only the phosphate and the active aldehyde group of the coenzyme. When taken in excess quantity, vitamin B$_6$ may be able to bind to some enzymes at their PLP binding sites and thereby inhibit the binding of the cofactor. This effect prevents the coenzyme from functioning, and thereby produces the same symptoms as a deficiency would. This phenomenon, whereby an excess of vitamin B$_6$ produces some of the same effects as its deficiency, was first discovered in a young woman who took excessive quantities of vitamin B$_6$ for menstrual cramps.

THE GABA SYNAPSE

Although synapses specialized for GABA have many biochemical similarities to those of other amino acid neurotransmitters, they also have some metabolic peculiarities. The astrocytes that surround every synapse play a specific role in GABA function.

Most amino acid neurotransmitters are functionally inactivated by re-uptake from the synaptic cleft into the presynaptic terminal. GABA, however, is taken up primarily by the glial cells associated with the synapse. Once inside the glial cell's mitochondria, GABA is transaminated by GABA-T and passes its amino group into a molecule of glutamate. GABA's carbon skeleton is then catabolized to carbon dioxide by the glial cell's citric acid cycle. This process involves the reactions shown in Figure 4-3.

The newly synthesized glutamate, containing the nitrogen from GABA, is next converted to glutamine by glutamine synthetase. Glutamine synthetase is relatively specific to glial cells, not being a neuronal enzyme. This reaction adds another nitrogen to the molecule, this time as an amide on a carboxyl group, and neutralizes the molecule. Glutamine, the product of this reaction, is electrostatically neutral, as it has both one positive and one negative charge. The glutamine migrates back to the presynaptic neuron, where glutaminase, an enzyme specific

Figure 4-3 Schematic Diagram of Flow of Neurotransmitter Molecules in a GABA-ergic Synapse

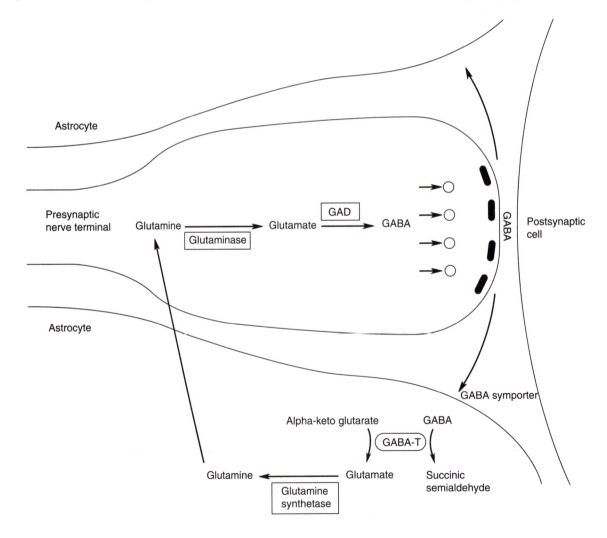

to neurons, converts it back into a molecule of glutamate. As glutamate, it is now able to reenter the GABA shunt.

Since the molecule taken up by the glial cell contains four carbons and one nitrogen, and the molecule given off to the neuron contains five carbons and two nitrogens, a net transfer of one nitrogen and one carbon from an astrocyte to an adjacent neuron occurs for each molecule of GABA taken up by the glial cell. This process contains an energy advantage for the neuron, in that the TCA cycle in the neuron is left relatively intact and the reactions of the GABA shunt occur predominantly in glia. Astrocytes oxidize four carbon units and synthesize five carbon units, while the neuron continues producing three NADH for each turn of the citric acid cycle. This metabolic arrangement supports the notion of glial cells' having a supportive metabolic role for neurons.

SELF-STUDY QUESTIONS

Facts:

1. Which amino acids are used as excitatory transmitters and which as inhibitory transmitters?

2. What are the ion permeability effects of glutamate, GABA, and glycine?

3. What are the synaptic inactivation mechanisms for glutamate, GABA, and glycine?

Concepts:

1. Describe the evolutionary advantage of amino acid transmitters being non-essential amino acids.

2. Define receptor degeneracy.

3. Discuss the functional significance of the glutamate/GABA ratio and its potential effects on CNS irritability.

4. Describe the mechanism of the metabolic response to hypoxia and hypoglycemia and its effect on amino acid transmitters.

5. Describe the mechanism of seizure susceptibility with a deficiency of pyridoxine.

6. Describe the mechanism of the neuronal advantage from glial cell metabolism of GABA.

BIBLIOGRAPHY

McGeer, P.L., Eccles, J.C., and McGeer, E.G. 1987. *Molecular Neurobiology of the Mammalian Brain*, 2nd ed. New York: Plenum Press.

CHAPTER 5

Acetylcholine

Acetylcholine (Ach, Figure 5-1), along with norepinephrine (NE, or noradrenaline), is the earliest-known neurotransmitter. Both are active in the autonomic nervous system as well as in the central nervous system (CNS). Neither, however, is the transmitter found in greatest quantity within the CNS. Acetylcholine is predominantly located in (1) the septum, which supplies acetylcholine to the septal-hippocampal tract; (2) the nucleus basalis of Meynert, located in the prefrontal forebrain; (3) the Renshaw **interneurons** in the spinal cord; and (4) interneurons within the striatum. Although the total amount of Ach is small in CNS, it may be particularly important in some motor functions and in higher mentation, such as learning.

SYNTHESIS

The **choline** transporter from blood is half saturated at a choline concentration of about 1 μM (i.e., the Km is 1 μM). Therefore, whatever choline is present in blood will be efficiently transported into CNS. The amount of choline in blood is highly variable, depending on many factors but especially on the amount of choline in recent meals. Choline is consumed in the diet primarily as phosphatidyl choline (PC), the major phospholipid in most eukaryotic membranes. A meal rich in PC has been shown to raise the blood concentration of choline for a few hours thereafter.

The synthesis of Ach is catalyzed by choline acetyl transferase (ChAT), which creates the ester bond using acetyl CoA and free choline as substrates. In brain, the acetyl group comes from the metabolism of glucose. There are two major sources of free choline. Most choline used for Ach synthesis comes from the bloodstream, with the aid of the transporter across the blood–brain barrier. A smaller pool of choline comes from endogenous synthesis. This latter process does not synthesize choline directly. Instead, phosphatidyl choline is made from

Figure 5-1
Acetylcholine

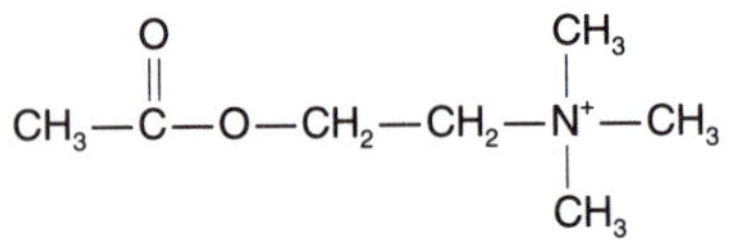

$$CH_3-\overset{\overset{\displaystyle O}{\|}}{C}-O-CH_2-CH_2-\overset{\overset{\displaystyle CH_3}{|}}{\underset{\underset{\displaystyle CH_3}{|}}{N^+}}-CH_3$$

phosphatidyl ethanolamine or phosphatidyl serine. The choline residue may subsequently be released from the lipid by hydrolysis.

Choline acetyl transferase has a Km for choline of about 1 mM, which is fairly high compared to Kms of similar enzymes for their substrates. The importance of an enzyme's Km is well illustrated in the case of choline, as the normal concentration of choline in brain tissue is considerably below 1 mM, normally about 10–20 μM. If 1 mM choline is required for half saturation of the enzyme, 20 μM will provide less than 1 percent saturation. In such a situation, significant changes in the substrate concentration will produce large changes in the activity of the enzyme; in effect, the enzyme is controlled by the substrate concentration rather than by allosteric mechanisms. As a general principle, when an enzyme's Km for a substrate is much higher than the steady state concentration of that substrate, the enzyme's activity is controlled by substrate concentration.

Therefore, modest changes of available choline can result in large changes in the amount of Ach being made. As discussed earlier, transmitter release from an axon terminal is proportional to the amount of calcium mobilized in the cytoplasm, but the calcium does not effect release of transmitter molecules directly. Calcium makes possible the membrane fusion events necessary for releasing the contents of synaptic vesicles. Therefore, changes in the amount of transmitter being stored in the vesicles will result in changes in the amount of transmitter released per nerve impulse. If more Ach is synthesized as a result of an increase in available choline, more will be released into the cleft. In this way, it is possible for the blood level of choline, as determined by dietary intake, to determine the functional status of brain Ach.

This arrangement, whereby dietary levels of a substrate can regulate brain synaptic function, is true of at least three neurotransmitters: acetylcholine, serotonin, and histamine. The fact that diet controls the function of any neuro-transmitter is of significance and suggests a potential site for therapeutic intervention. In the case of Ach, although there is controversy about it, there is evidence that elevated blood choline, induced by adding PC to the diet, results in increased Ach synthesis and release from its terminals. Adding PC to the diet has been tried as a treatment for several neurological diseases in which a loss of Ach has been found, including Alzheimer's disease. The success of this approach is questionable, however.

SYNAPTIC DYNAMICS

Ach is stored in vesicles with vesiculin, the name given its storage glycosaminoglycan. ChAT may be associated with the cytoplasmic surface of the vesicle membrane, where the product of its reaction (Ach) would have immediate access to the vesicle's Ach transporter, and thereby to its storage mechanism.

Acetylcholine receptors are usually classified into muscarinic and **nicotinic,** according to which plant alkaloid, either muscarine or nicotine, activates the receptor. Muscarinic receptors are slow acting and are more prominent in brain than are nicotinic receptors. Muscarinic receptors are indirect, or second messenger, receptors and are now known to have multiple subclasses. The receptors from several different tracts have been isolated and **cloned,** and at least five different amino acid sequences have been found in them, all of which are within the rhodopsin family of receptors (see Chapter 11).

Nicotinic receptors, the predominant acetylcholine receptor at the myoneural junction (i.e., nerve endings on muscle cells), are fast acting and are less common in brain. Nicotinic receptors belong to the class we are calling direct receptors, and are ion channels (see Chapter 9).

Both muscarinic and nicotinic receptors are usually classified as producing epsp's. Nicotinic receptors are "all-ion" depolarizing channels when activated by the presence of Ach. Muscarinic receptors often produce an epsp by diminishing a K^+ ion current, and use second messengers to accomplish this (Chapter 11). Since increasing K^+ permeability produces hyperpolarization, decreasing it is classified as an epsp. Some muscarinic receptors also have been reported to lower the concentration of **cAMP,** raise **cGMP,** and/or increase the production of **nitric oxide** (NO) (Chapter 11). Several are known to be linked to the phosphatidyl inositide "second messenger" system. So, despite the fact that Ach is not found in many tracts and is not a major transmitter in terms of its concentration in whole brain, its functions are neurologically important and it exemplifies the complexity of neurotransmitter receptor systems.

SYNAPTIC INACTIVATION

The action of Ach is stopped within the synaptic cleft by catabolism, specifically with hydrolysis by the enzyme acetylcholinesterase (AchE). AchE is a membrane-anchored enzyme, being attached to the extracellular side of synaptic membranes by a link to a phospholipid (phosphatidyl inositol), similar to the anchoring of the $5'$ nucleotidase of glia. AchE appears to be found on all the membranes, glial and neuronal, in cholinergic synapses. AchE is rather common, being present in many places within the CNS where neither Ach nor its synthetic enzyme, ChAT, is found. Attempts to localize the site of action of Ach by histochemical determination of AchE have not been completely reliable for this reason, whereas the localization of ChAT is a consistent indicator for the distribution of Ach.

RECYCLING

Whereas the transmitter is inactivated in the cleft by AchE, the choline itself can be reused. Presynaptic terminals of cholinergic neurons have a choline transporter, which serves to recycle most residual choline back into the terminal, where it can be used to make more Ach. This mechanism also has an effect on function, as outlined above. As the synapse works faster, larger amounts of choline may be available in the cleft, from the hydrolysis of lipids as well as of Ach. This means that larger amounts become available in the terminal, which in turn means that more Ach will be synthesized. This is a kind of positive feed forward mechanism, allowing a significant up regulation of cholinergic synapses, in response to a long-term activation.

As long as free choline is present in the cleft, and especially if the concentration is high, it may continue to activate muscarinic receptors. Its binding constant (K_D) is much higher than that of Ach, so it takes a higher concentration to be effective, but large amounts of choline can produce cholinergic activation. Activation may occur during conditions of high Ach turnover; it could also occur during unusually high phospholipid turnover in the membrane.

As mentioned above, Ach is not found in large quantity in brain, but several cholinergic tracts have been identified. Ach has been postulated to play a role in many CNS functions, from regulation of blood flow to higher learning, but most of these hypotheses are not yet definitive. Some of the most heavily studied cholinergic areas include tracts from the septum to the **hippocampus** and from the nucleus basalis to the cortex. These may be involved in learning. A group of cholinergic neurons in the **brainstem,** in conjunction with serotonergic and noradrenergic cells, is involved in the regulation of sleep cycles.

SELF-STUDY QUESTIONS

Facts:

1. What enzyme synthesizes Ach, and what are its substrates?

2. Where are Ach tracts located within the CNS?

3. What are the kinds of Ach receptors, and which is predominant?

4. What method of synaptic inactivation is used for Ach?

5. What method is used for recycling choline?

6. How is Ach stored in its synaptic vesicles?

Concepts:

1. Describe the circumstances under which substrate concentration controls transmitter expression.

2. Discuss dietary intervention strategies for Ach.

BIBLIOGRAPHY

Blusztajn, J.K., and Wurtman, R.J. 1983. Choline and cholinergic neurons. *Science* 221: 614–620.

Taylor, P., and Brown, J.H. 1989. Acetylcholine. In *Basic Neurochemistry*, edited by G. Siegel, B. Agranoff, R.W. Albers, and P. Molinoff. New York: Raven Press.

CHAPTER 6

Catecholamine Neurotransmitters

Catechol is the name given an aromatic ring with two hydroxyl groups attached to adjacent carbons (Figure 6-1). The catecholamine neurotransmitters have hydroxyl groups in the 3 and 4 positions of the ring. The number 4 carbon is opposite the side chain. The neighboring carbon with a hydroxyl group is carbon number 3. All three catecholamines found in the CNS (dopamine, DA; noradrenaline, or norepinephrine, NE; and adrenaline, or epinephrine, EPI) are present in small concentrations overall, although their functions are quite important.

Epinephrine is not usually present in discrete nuclei. The neurons that use it as a transmitter are distributed among several areas of the brain. It is difficult to study a transmitter that is found in multiple sites in low concentration. Therefore, compared to DA and NE, not as much is known about EPI and its function in the CNS, although its CNS metabolism can be studied. Neurons that use DA and NE as transmitters, on the other hand, are localized. DA and NE are usually thought of as transmitters of arousal, as increasing their activity is associated with increased activity of the whole organism.

Increased DA activity is associated with increased physical activity and with different kinds of psychological arousal and it is involved in the experience of pleasure.

Dopaminergic neurons are found in highest concentration in the substantia nigra, whence most axons innervate the neostriatum (i.e., the nigrostriatal tract). Two small nuclei associated with the substantia nigra (designated A9 and A10) are also dopaminergic. These are sometimes called the ventral tegmental area (VTA). These two smaller groups of neurons form the mesocortical/mesolimbic system— that is, they are located in the **mesencephalon** and they send axonal processes to the **cortex** and the **limbic system.** The mesocortical/mesolimbic system is smaller and less clearly defined than the nigrostriatal tract and contains less total dopamine. It is, however, thought to be of considerable importance. The mesocortical/ mesolimbic system may play a central role in schizophrenia (Chapter 16) and may also play an important role in other states, such as manic-depressive psychosis (Chapter 17) and addiction to drugs such as cocaine and amphetamines (Chapter 13).

NE is localized within the CNS to an even more striking degree than DA. Essentially all CNS NE exists in the neurons of the locus ceruleus (LC). This nucleus, limited to a few tens or hundreds of thousands of cell bodies, innervates

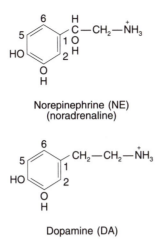

Norepinephrine (NE)
(noradrenaline)

Dopamine (DA)

**Figure 6-1 Two
Catecholamine
Neurotransmitters**

much of the rest of the CNS. Therefore, NE is found throughout much of the brain, but in very small quantities. The LC is functionally important in pleasure (as well as its opposite, anxiety) and in learning and sleep (see below). It is often thought of as a system primarily involved in psychological arousal, attention, or focus, whereas dopamine is more heavily involved in motor arousal.

TRANSPORT

The synthesis of catecholamines begins with the amino acid tyrosine. Tyrosine is not usually listed as an essential amino acid because the human body is capable of synthesizing it from phenylalanine. But the enzyme required for the synthesis, phenylalanine hydroxylase, is a liver enzyme that is not found in brain. Therefore, the brain cannot make tyrosine and it is as dependent upon a steady supply of tyrosine from the bloodstream as it is for all of the essential amino acids. Thus, from the standpoint of the CNS, tyrosine is an essential amino acid.

This fact is of significance primarily because of the transporter required for tyrosine's entry into CNS. The transporter, the large neutral amino acid transporter (LNAA), is located in the vascular epithelium and transports several essential amino acids from blood, in addition to tyrosine. The most important substrates for the LNAA are tyrosine, phenylalanine, tryptophan, methionine, valine, leucine, and isoleucine. Since none of these can be synthesized in brain, all are required by brain for the synthesis of normal brain proteins. Tyrosine and tryptophan are required in extra quantity (beyond that necessary for protein synthesis) because they are also precursors for neurotransmitters. Methionine is also required in extra quantities, as it is a major source of methyl groups for the synthesis of phosphatidyl choline and for the metabolism of some transmitters.

Because a single transporter is used for all of these necessary amino acids, the substrates in effect compete with each other for entry across the blood–brain barrier into the CNS. If the pattern, or ratio, of LNAA substrates is altered, the distribution of amino acids entering the CNS will be skewed. This imbalance may create a deficiency in one or more necessary amino acids. Such an imbalance is one of the proposed explanations for certain types of mental retardation, such as maple syrup urine disease and phenylketonuria. If phenylalanine, for example, builds up in high concentration in blood, due to a deficiency of phenylalanine hydroxylase in liver, its excess concentration could prevent adequate amounts of methionine, tryptophan, valine, isoleucine, and leucine from entering the CNS. Such a state could lead to a deficiency of transmitters and other molecules (i.e., proteins and lipids) synthesized from these essential substrates.

ANABOLISM

Under normal circumstances, the LNAA transports tyrosine into the CNS in more than adequate quantity. Therefore, tyrosine is usually not rate limiting for the synthesis of catecholamines. The first enzyme of the pathway, tyrosine hydroxylase (TH), is an allosterically regulated, rate-limiting enzyme. TH is a monooxygenase, a type of enzyme that requires molecular oxygen and a reducing agent as **stoichiometric** cosubstrates, in addition to the molecule being hydroxylated. In the case of TH, tyrosine receives a hydroxyl (OH) group, and tetrahydrobiopterin (THB) is the reducing agent. An Fe^{++} is also required by the enzyme as a catalytic cofactor (i.e., a coenzyme required in equal amount to the enzyme). The products of the reaction are dihydroxyphenylalanine (DOPA), H_2O, and dihydrobiopterin (DHB) (Figure 6-2). During the reaction, one molecule of tyrosine is oxidized (by hydroxylation), one atom of oxygen is reduced to water, and one molecule of THB is oxidized to DHB (by dehydrogenation). The DHB must be rereduced by another enzyme before it is again usable.

TH is allosterically regulated. DA, and possibly NE, bind to the inhibitory allosteric site when their concentrations are high in the immediate vicinity of the enzyme. When this allosteric site is occupied, the enzymatic reaction is inhibited by elevation of the Km for THB (not for tyrosine). As the Km is raised, THB binds less well and, therefore, more THB is required to achieve the same rate of synthesis. This arrangement, whereby the binding of the cofactor is regulated, rather than the primary substrate (tyrosine), has the effect of introducing another regulatory mechanism into the activity of TH. Brain tyrosine levels are rarely rate limiting for TH, but THB is often rate limiting (Figure 6-3).

THB is a member of a class of molecules called pteridines (from the Greek *pteron*, meaning "wing," so called because they were first isolated from butterflies). THB has a ring structure similar to the vitamin folic acid. THB, however, is not a vitamin. It is synthesized within the cells that use it, meaning within those cells that contain any one of the four mammalian enzymes that require THB as a stoichiometric cofactor (i.e., cosubstrates).

Figure 6-2 The Tyrosine Hydroxylase Reaction

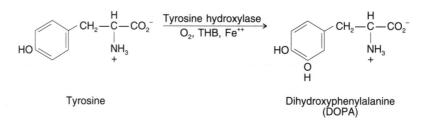

Tyrosine

Dihydroxyphenylalanine
(DOPA)

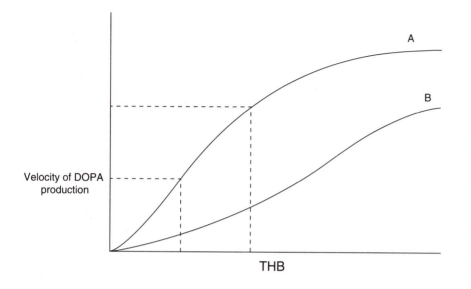

Figure 6-3 The allosteric regulation of tyrosine hydroxylase. *A is the activity curve in the presence of baseline levels of DA. B is the activity curve in the presence of a higher concentration of DA. In the latter case (curve B), a higher concentration of THB is required to achieve the same velocity of reaction.*

THB is synthesized in amounts such that its concentration is rate limiting when the enzyme is allosterically inhibited and saturating when the allosteric site is empty. As a result of these characteristics, biopterin derivatives can be used as potential interventions in cases in which greater synthesis of catecholamines is desired; supplementation with some biopterins (or molecules that can substitute for them) can in some cases increase the synthesis of catecholamine transmitters and thereby increase their function. Several other pteridine molecules seem to be able to affect the activity of tyrosine hydroxylase. For example, folic acid, which has a similar structure, may be able to increase TH activity, and is a possible intervention. Drugs that are similar in structure to pteridines (e.g., some diuretics) may also have CNS effects from interference with TH. This is an area for further study.

After TH, the next step in catecholamine transmitter synthesis is the decarboxylation of DOPA to dopamine (Figure 6-4). This enzyme is often called dopa decarboxylase, but it is more accurately referred to as aromatic amino acid decarboxylase (AAAD), because of its lack of specificity for substrate and its occurrence in different neurons. AAAD, as is true of other amino acid decarboxylases, requires pyridoxal phosphate (PLP) as a cofactor. Again, in common with other amino acid decarboxylases, it must bind to the concentration of PLP in the intracellular pool. This implies that the enzyme has a separate binding site for PLP and a specific Km for it, analogous to the binding of THB to TH (Figure 6-2).

As mentioned above, in vivo AAAD is found in many different cells and has multiple substrates. It is usually present in sufficient quantity that its activity is not

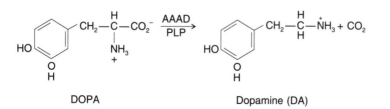

Figure 6-4 The aromatic amino acid decarboxylase (AAAD) reaction. *AAAD is sometimes called DOPA decarboxylase.*

rate limiting for the synthesis of any of the transmitters in which it is involved. It is theoretically possible, of course, for the enzyme to be sufficiently inhibited or to be so low in concentration that it becomes a rate-limiting factor. It also could be inhibited by a deficiency of vitamin B_6, from which PLP is made. In certain situations, inhibition of AAAD could also be a cause of mental retardation. Further data related to this possibility are discussed in Chapter 12. In dopaminergic cells, TH and AAAD are sufficient to synthesize the cells' transmitters. In these cells, DA is then transported into synaptic vesicles, where it is stored prior to release. In noradrenergic cells, the same transport and storage of DA take place, but the final synthetic step occurs in the synaptic vesicle (Figure 6-5).

Dopamine beta-hydroxylase (DBH) is sequestered in the vesicles of neurons containing noradrenaline and adrenaline. It is also a monooxygenase, requiring a metal ion, oxygen, and a reducing agent. DBH uses neither Fe^{++} nor THB. The metal in this case is Cu^{++}, and the reducing, stoichiometric cofactor is ascorbate (vitamin C). DBH is also an allosteric enzyme, regulated by the amount of NE in the vesicle. Therefore, there are two levels of allosteric regulation of NE synthesis. One is in the cytoplasm, where DA inhibits TH, and the other is in the synaptic vesicle, where NE inhibits DBH.

In cells that use adrenaline, or epinephrine (EPI), as transmitter, a final synthetic step is necessary. The NE produced by DBH is methylated, forming EPI. The methylating enzyme, phenylethanolamine N-methyltransferase (PNMT), uses **S-adenosyl methionine (SAM)** as a donor for the methyl group it attaches to NE (Figure 6-5). PNMT, as the final enzyme for EPI synthesis, is specific for EPI. Its location correlates with the use of EPI as a transmitter, and it is distributed in many places throughout the CNS. Neurons using EPI as a transmitter are widespread, with many in the cerebral cortex.

Also within the synaptic vesicle—along with the transmitter, ATP, metal ions, and (in the case of a noradrenergic synapse) DBH—there is a storage (glyco-) protein. This glycosaminoglycan, discussed in Chapter 3, is necessary for osmotic reasons. The storage protein in noradrenergic cells is called chromogranin A, and that in dopaminergic cells is called chromogranin B. The levels of some of these molecules can be useful for clinical purposes, in that their concentrations in bodily fluids reflect the amount of presynaptic activity of the transmitter over the previous several days. For example, synaptic release of NE allows a small amount of both DBH and chromogranin A to escape from the terminal as well. These large protein molecules are not catabolized as readily in extracellular fluid as transmitters are, and consequently are found in both CSF and blood. The levels of both molecules in CSF are proportional to the average amount of release of NE from its terminals in CNS over the previous period of hours to days. The same is true for chromogranin B from DA cells.

Although it is possible to measure these molecules in blood, since they must leave CSF and enter the bloodstream, their concentration there is much less useful

Figure 6-5 The Hydroxylation of DA to Make Noradrenaline (Norepinephrine)

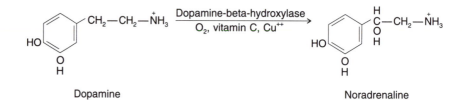

Dopamine   Noradrenaline

for neurological purposes than their concentration in CSF. The reason for this is the large amount of NE, epinephrine, and even some DA released from the adrenal medulla into blood. Since the peripheral turnover of catecholamines is far larger in the adrenal medulla than it is in brain, blood levels of these ancillary molecules predominantly reflect peripheral activity.

SYNAPTIC SPECIFICS

Catecholaminergic synapses have autoreceptors (on the axon terminal) as well as postsynaptic receptors. The most common dopamine autoreceptors are D2, and those for norepinephrine are α 2. The most common postsynaptic receptors are D1 and β 2, respectively. The autoreceptors, D2 and α 2, are both often associated with adenylyl cyclase within the cell of origin, where they inhibit the enzyme and reduce the production of cAMP. This inhibitory effect is often achieved through a **Gi** protein (see Chapter 11). The reduction in cAMP levels lessens the likelihood of further release of transmitter, so this mechanism functions as a kind of negative feedback regulation (NFB) for the terminal.

The common postsynaptic receptors for DA and NE, D1 and β 2, are also usually associated with cAMP production, but in the opposite direction: cAMP is increased. The postsynaptic effect of DA or NE, when released directly onto brain cells, is usually inhibitory, making the cells less likely to produce an action potential. Since both transmitters usually increase cAMP levels in postsynaptic cells, it may be that cAMP is often an inhibitory second messenger. This point is not entirely clear, however. The full effects of transmitters' second messenger activity are not entirely known.

One important implication of the above observations is the dissociation between the effects a transmitter produces at the cellular level and the effects it produces at the level of the whole organism. If the above facts are indeed true, then both dopamine and noradrenaline produce an arousal of the entire organism, and do so by inhibiting their postsynaptic cells. For this to be the case, many of the postsynaptic cells for catecholamine transmitters must themselves be inhibitory cells. Therefore, organismic arousal could arise from inhibiting inhibitory functions. This fundamental concept of disinhibition, as discussed earlier, appears in fact to be a common theme of brain function. The effects of DA and NE are examples of disinhibition at the cellular and organ level. It has been proposed that most brain synapses are inhibitory and that most "activation" actually occurs by some kind of disinhibition process.

As more brain tracts and pathways become known, it is clear that in order to understand whether a particular tract is inhibitory or excitatory, one must determine the number of inhibitory and excitatory neurons in the entire pathway, and how many of each are in sequence. An even number of successive inhibitory cells results in an excitatory effect; an odd number produces inhibition.

CATABOLISM

After their release into the synaptic cleft, catecholamines act upon autoreceptors and then upon postsynaptic receptors. They are also subjected to the influences of both extracellular enzymes and membrane transporters. Although the most important mechanism of physiological inactivation of catecholamine neurotransmitters is re-uptake into the presynaptic terminal, these molecules also must be catabolized over time. Some catabolism occurs both in the extracellular fluid of the synaptic cleft and within cells. Catabolism of catecholamines usually begins in the cleft, where catechol-O-methyl transferase (COMT) methylates the hydroxyl group at position 3 (Figures 6-6 and 6-7). S-adenosyl methionine (SAM) is the source of the methyl group, as it apparently has access to the extracellular enzyme. COMT is most likely anchored to the membranes around the cleft by a lipid-inositol anchor.

The resulting methylated molecule, called normetanephrine in the case of noradrenaline, for example, retains a small amount of activity at noradrenaline's receptors. Therefore, this extracellular enzymatic reaction is not a complete inactivation. The Na^+-coupled transporter (symporter) on the presynaptic plasma membrane is able to transport either the catecholamine or the 3-methyl derivative back into the cytoplasmic compartment. Similar transporters in the plasma membrane of nearby cells may account for some transmitter uptake, as well.

Once inside the cytoplasmic compartment, the catecholamine is a substrate for at least two competing processes. It can either be retransported into a synaptic vesicle or be acted upon by monoamine oxidase (MAO). MAO is a membrane enzyme attached to the outer membrane of mitochondria. It is oriented such that it works upon substrate molecules in the cytoplasm. MAO removes the amino group from the carbon to which it is attached and oxidizes that carbon to an aldehyde in the process. This eliminates any transmitter activity, as well as generating a (potentially) toxic aldehyde group.

Non-specific aldehyde oxidases or reductases then either oxidize the aldehyde to an acid or reduce it to an **alcohol.** In either case, the molecule is less

Figure 6-6 The Catabolism of Dopamine

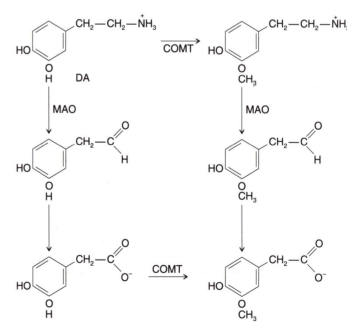

Homovanillic acid (HVA)

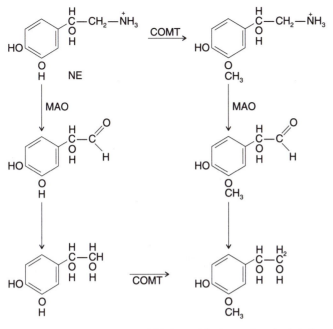

3-Methoxy-4-hydroxy-phenyl ethyl glycol (MHPG)

**Figure 6-7 The
Catabolism of
Norepinephrine (NE)**

toxic than a free aldehyde. In the metabolism of catecholamines, the order of
catabolic enzymes does not affect the structure of the final end products. If the
transmitter begins catabolism in the extracellular fluid, being methylated by
COMT, the methylated derivative loses its amino group within a cell later. If MAO
oxidizes the transmitter first, the products will later be methylated outside the cell.
The final products of these processes for the two major catecholamine transmitters
are of clinical interest, because their measurement in CSF provides an indication of
transmitter changes in disease states.

The final end product of dopamine catabolism is homovanillic acid (HVA,
4-hydroxy-3-methoxy-phenyl acetate) (Figure 6-6). In this case, the aldehyde
produced by MAO is oxidized to the corresponding acid. HVA levels in CSF have
been measured and shown to correlate with pathology. For example, HVA levels
are below normal in the CSF of Parkinson's disease patients, who have suffered a
loss of dopaminergic cells.

The catabolism of noradrenaline most frequently takes a different path. The
aldehyde produced by MAO is usually reduced in the CNS, not oxidized.
Therefore, the final product of noradrenaline metabolism in brain is 4-hydroxy-3-
methoxy-phenyl ethyl glycol (MHPG) (Figure 6-7). The productiveness of
attempts to find correlations between MHPG and various disease states is
questionable. MHPG levels in blood, and possibly in CSF, vary somewhat with
the time of day in which the measurement is taken and possibly in response to other
environmental factors such as diet and exercise. There is some evidence, however,
that levels of MHPG are elevated in CSF during the manic phase of manic-
depressive psychosis. There is a possible correlation, somewhat less clear,
between MHPG and certain aspects of schizophrenia, as well.

SELF-STUDY QUESTIONS

Facts:

1. What are the major dopaminergic and noradrenergic tracts?

2. What functions are DA and NE usually associated with at the level of the whole organism?

3. What cellular changes are usually produced by DA and NE?

4. What receptor mechanisms are usually used by DA and NE?

5. How are DA and NE inactivated after synaptic release?

6. Where are the enzymes of synthesis for DA and NE?

7. Where are the enzymes of catabolism for DA and NE?

Concepts:

1. Predict the effects of antagonists at each of the macromolecular binding sites for DA and NE within the synapse.

2. Describe the methods of regulation of synthetic enzymes for DA and NE.

3. Discuss the relationship between levels of final catabolites of DA and NE and disease processes.

BIBLIOGRAPHY

Dohlman, H.G., Thorner, J., Caron, M.G., and Lefkowitz, R.J. 1991. Model systems for the study of seven-transmembrane-segment receptors. *Annual Review of Biochemistry* 60: 653–688.

Moore, R.Y., and Bloom, F.E. 1978. Central catecholamine neuron systems: Anatomy and physiology of the dopamine systems. *Annual Review of Neuroscience* 1: 129–169.

Moore, R.Y., and Bloom, F.E. 1979. Central catecholamine neuron systems: Anatomy and physiology of the norepinephrine and epinephrine systems. *Annual Review of Neuroscience* 2: 113–168.

CHAPTER 7

Serotonin and the Pineal Body

SEROTONIN

Serotonin is also called 5-hydroxytryptamine, or 5-HT. Nearly all the serotonin in the CNS is located within the neurons of the Raphe nuclei, which are spread along the midline of the pons. These neurons have a "sprinkler system" arrangement of axons that provides serotonergic innervation to much of the rest of the CNS, even to the spinal cord, much as do the axon projections from the locus ceruleus and the mesolimbic/mesocortical system.

Serotonin, in common with the catecholamines, is synthesized within the brain from an essential amino acid, for which the brain is dependent upon the blood for its supply. Serotonin's precursor, tryptophan, is carried across the blood–brain barrier by the large neutral amino acid transporter (LNAA), which also carries tyrosine for synthesis of catecholamines (see Chapter 6). Since neither tyrosine nor any of the other essential amino acids can be synthesized in brain, a continuous supply of these amino acids from blood is necessary.

The rate-limiting enzyme of serotonin's synthesis is tryptophan hydroxylase (TRPH), and its kinetic characteristics are similar to those of choline acetyl transferase (see Chapter 5). This means that its Km for tryptophan is higher than the usual concentration of tryptophan within the brain. Therefore, in most circumstances, the concentration of tryptophan is the rate-limiting factor for the synthesis of serotonin. This fact implies that, as with acetylcholine and histamine, blood levels of the precursor control the brain's functional levels of a transmitter. Although it is true that blood concentrations of tryptophan can regulate brain serotonin function, the circumstances are more complex in this case than with histamine and acetylcholine. Tryptophan's ability to control serotonin synthesis is also affected by other factors, specifically, the presence of other amino acids in the blood and the carbohydrate content of meals.

Tryptophan is the most limited amino acid in foodstuffs, and indeed, in all of biology. Its concentration is therefore small compared to other substrates for the LNAA. The LNAA responds to the ratio, or pattern, of concentrations of substrate amino acids in the bloodstream. It transports amino acids according to that pattern, and according to each amino acid's ability to bind the transporter. This characteristic means that significant changes in the concentration in blood of one or more of the substrates of the LNAA will cause major changes in what is transported. In other words, the amount of tryptophan transported across the blood–brain barrier is determined in part by the concentration of tryptophan in blood and in part by the concentration of the other amino acids that compete with it. In practice, the three branched-chain hydrophobic amino acids, leucine (L), isoleucine (I), and valine (V), are the most crucial competitors with tryptophan (W). A rough correlation of the extent of tryptophan transport into brain is given by the ratio in blood of tryptophan concentration to the total concentrations of L, I, and V (W/L + V + I).

The transport of tryptophan by the LNAA, and therefore the synthesis of serotonin, is sensitive to carbohydrate consumption. The transport and synthesis depend on the fact that the concentration of the branched-chain amino acids in blood is affected by insulin activity. Branched-chain amino acids, especially leucine, both respond to insulin and serve as signals to stimulate insulin secretion. Glucose works in a similar way. Thus, when a person eats a meal containing both carbohydrate and amino acids, insulin secretion is increased. This is in response to both glucose and leucine, as well as other factors. The increased insulin concentration in blood then results in a decrease in leucine, isoleucine, and valine, as well as glucose, because insulin increases the transport of these molecules into muscle and other tissues. It has been observed that blood tryptophan levels are unaffected by insulin. Therefore, the ratio of tryptophan to the other LNAA substrates is greatly increased when the above-mentioned molecules are transported to muscle and other tissues. The higher ratio of tryptophan results in increased transport of tryptophan into CNS and increased serotonin synthesis. This in turn increases serotonin's CNS effects. One such effect is increased sleepiness, as serotonin is an inhibitor of arousal. This phenomenon is often cited as the cause of the drowsiness that people commonly experience after lunch.

Supplementing one's diet with tryptophan, as many people do, will raise the ratio of blood tryptophan to I, L, and V and increase the transport of tryptophan into the CNS. In some people, this has a tranquilizing effect. Supplementing the diet with other substrates of the LNAA will lower the amount of tryptophan transported into the CNS. There are hazards to such supplementation, however. Some commercial preparations of tryptophan contain toxic contaminants, and these contaminants have recently been implicated as the cause of a bone marrow disease in several people who took the supplement in high doses. Additionally, increasing the relative concentrations of one amino acid (especially tryptophan) compared to other amino acids can have toxic effects on the liver.

These facts regarding the kinetics of the LNAA and its effect on serotonin synthesis also help explain some of the pathology of certain genetic diseases. Phenylketonuria (PKU) is a disease caused by the deficiency of phenylalanine hydroxylase, a liver enzyme. Because of the deficiency of this enzyme, its substrate, phenylalanine (abbreviated F), builds up in blood. Phenylalanine is one of the molecules that compete with tryptophan for the LNAA; as a result of the buildup of phenylalanine, tryptophan transport into CNS is diminished. This results in decreased serotonin synthesis. A similar situation occurs in maple syrup urine disease (MSUD), in which deaminated derivatives of I, V, and L build up in blood and compete with tryptophan transport.

Anabolism

The enzyme affected by tryptophan concentrations is tryptophan hydroxylase (TRPH). This enzyme is in many ways analogous to tyrosine hydroxylase (TH) (involved in the synthesis of catecholamines; see Chapter 6), especially regarding its mechanism of action. It is a monooxygenase, requiring molecular oxygen, tetrahydrobiopterin (THB), and ferrous iron (Fe^{++}), in addition to tryptophan. It is analogous to TH in that the cells that contain TRPH also make their own THB, but TRPH is different in that THB is apparently not the rate-limiting factor. Whereas tyrosine concentration is rarely rate limiting for TH activity, tryptophan concentration appears to be the primary regulator of TRPH activity. The Km of tryptophan for TRPH is about 300 μM, which is much greater than the normal steady-state concentration of tryptophan in brain (about 10 μM). Thus, small changes in intracellular neuronal tryptophan concentration can cause large changes in the amount of serotonin synthesized. This, in turn, causes a significant increase in serotonin released when neurons in the Raphe nucleus are activated. This is similar to the situation observed in acetylcholine synthesis. The ability of supplementary tryptophan to increase serotonin synthesis is much greater than the ability of choline to increase Ach synthesis, however. In lower animals, it has been shown that brain serotonin can be increased up to tenfold by adding tryptophan in the diet. This is probably the greatest such dietary effect for any neurotransmitter.

The next step in serotonin synthesis (following the tryptophan hydroxylase–catalyzed reaction) is catalyzed by essentially the same enzyme found in catecholaminergic cells, aromatic amino acid decarboxylase (AAAD), using pyridoxal phosphate (PLP) as a cofactor. This enzyme is sometimes called dopa decarboxylase. The product of TRPH, 5-hydroxytryptophan, is a substrate for AAAD, which converts it into serotonin (Figure 7-1). One transporter and two enzymes thus transform serum tryptophan into the neurotransmitter serotonin. In serotonergic cells, AAAD may be associated with the cytoplasmic surface of synaptic vesicles. Such a location assures that the transmitter, the product of the reaction, has immediate access to the vesicular transporter and to storage in presynaptic vesicles.

The transporter used in the vesicular membrane may be the same one used in catecholaminergic synapses. Evidence for this is provided by the observation that the drug reserpine has the same effect on dopamine and noradrenaline that it has on serotonin. Reserpine binds the vesicular transporter and irreversibly inhibits it, preventing the transmitter from leaving the cytoplasm and entering the vesicles. As serotonin's concentration rises in cytoplasm, much of it is catabolized to inactive products by monoamine oxidase (MAO). Therefore, reserpine leads to the depletion of catecholamines and serotonin from the cells that use them as transmitters, thus decreasing their effects within the CNS.

Serotonergic Effects

The Raphe nuclei innervate much of the CNS, thus providing widespread effects. At the level of the whole organism, serotonin's effect is normally a

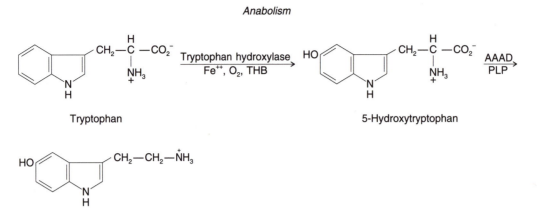

Anabolism

Tryptophan   5-Hydroxytryptophan

HO—[indole]—CH_2—CH_2—$\overset{+}{N}H_3$

Serotonin (5-hydroxytryptamine, 5-HT)

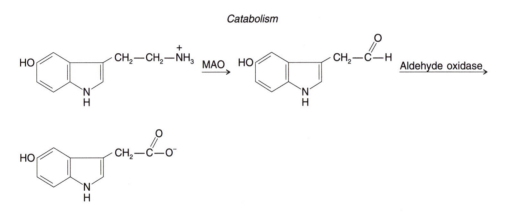

Catabolism

5-Hydroxy indole acetic acid (5-HIAA)

Figure 7-1 The Metabolism of Serotonin

diminished state of arousal. For example, increasing serotonin's synaptic activity causes an increase in total sleep time, an increase in slow-wave sleep time, and a decrease in sexual activity. Sexual activity is also decreased during wakefulness; it is not simply inhibited by the animal's spending more time asleep.

As is the case with catecholamine transmitters, serotonin's effect on postsynaptic cells and the effect on the organism may not be of the same kind. Catecholamines often inhibit their postsynaptic cells while activating or "arousing" the organism. Serotonin inhibits many of the organism's activities, while its postsynaptic effects may be mostly excitatory. The second messenger effects most commonly linked to serotonin receptors are thought to be excitatory. Serotonin may also exert its effects through intermediary inhibitory neurons.

Mechanism of Action

Once serotonin has been released from the presynaptic terminal, it binds and activates presynaptic, inhibitory receptors and postsynaptic receptors. It also may bind to, and be transported by, the re-uptake symporter on the presynaptic terminal. The two receptors and the transporter are pharmacologically distinct in that different drugs are **agonists** and **antagonists** for each. Lysergic acid diethylamide (LSD), for example, is an antagonist for several serotonin receptors, both presynaptic and postsynaptic. LSD appears to be fairly specific for serotonin receptors, but it also has some overlapping effects on catecholamine receptors, especially on those of noradrenaline.

The mechanism of LSD's action in producing hallucinations is thought to be predominantly a result of its effects on serotonergic synapses. This hypothesis is based, as well, on observations that implicate serotonin in visual phenomena, especially in dreaming. In lower animals, dreaming sleep can be determined by characteristic brain and muscle electrical activity. During these periods, electrical activity in the visual cortex that does not arise from the eyes, but instead comes from the brain stem, is observed. This activity may be originating from mono-aminergic cells in the brain stem. These patterns of electrical activity, called pontine-geniculate-occipital (PGO) spikes, also occur during LSD intoxication, as well as in other hallucinatory states.

Receptors

Serotonin has many different receptors, the structural details of which are being reported in the current scientific literature. Many serotonin receptors seem to function in mammals with second messengers from the phosphatidyl inositol system, rather than with adenylyl cyclase and cyclic AMP. In many invertebrates, where much of the research on serotonin's function has taken place, it is more commonly associated with the activation of adenylyl cyclase (see Chapter 12).

Catabolism

Serotonin is catabolized in only two steps, using monoamine oxidase (MAO) and a presumably non-specific aldehyde oxidase (Figure 7-1). MAO removes the amino nitrogen and oxidizes the carbon to which it was attached to an aldehyde. The aldehyde is then detoxified by further oxidation to an acid. The product of this reaction is 5-hydroxy indole acetic acid (5-HIAA), which is the final end product of serotonin metabolism in the CNS. It therefore is the molecule that leaves the CNS, moving from CSF into blood.

This catabolite is specific for serotonin, and therefore its levels in CSF may reflect CNS serotonin turnover. CSF levels of 5-HIAA have been correlated with disease states and are possible indicators of a serotonergic role in some psychiatric diseases, although there is some controversy about this interpretation. 5-HIAA has been studied most in schizophrenic and depressed patients. Serotonin levels have been found to be elevated in some situations indicating severe depression; for example, serotonin is increased in the brainstems of many suicide victims. 5-HIAA levels are similarly elevated in the CSF of many bipolar manic-depressive patients during their most depressed phase.

THE PINEAL BODY

The pineal body, or pineal gland, is situated immediately posterior to the hypothalamus, from which it differentiates during embryological growth. It is the richest animal source of serotonin, although the gland itself does not use serotonin as a transmitter. Within the pineal body, serotonin serves only as a substrate for the synthesis of the pineal's hormonal products (Figure 7-2). The most significant of these products is melatonin (from the Greek suffix *melas*, meaning "black"), named because it causes skin darkening in amphibians. Melatonin is an important mammalian hormone for regulating metabolic and behavioral changes in response to the cycle of the seasons. For example, both sexual activity and thermogenesis are significantly controlled by melatonin in some species. Melatonin is a potent inhibitor of the gonads in both sexes and a potent stimulator of brown adipose tissue (BAT), an organ specialized for heat production.

Synthesis of Melatonin

Melatonin's synthesis occurs in two steps, starting with a large pool of serotonin, which is maintained in pinealocytes. First, an N-acetyl transferase

Figure 7-2 The Synthesis of Hormones Within Pinealocytes

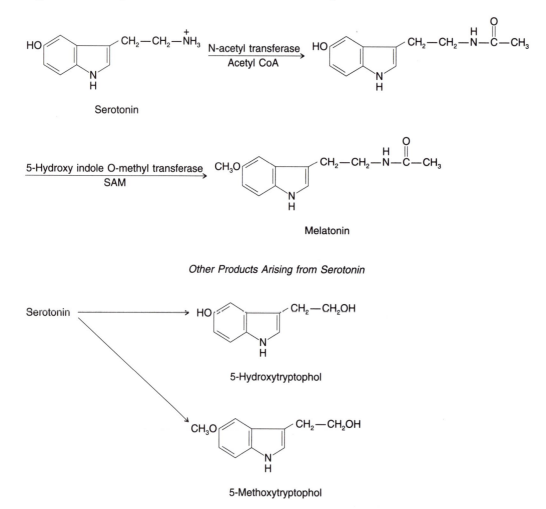

Serotonin

Melatonin

Other Products Arising from Serotonin

5-Hydroxytryptophol

5-Methoxytryptophol

(NAT) attaches an acetyl group, from acetyl CoA, to the nitrogen atom of serotonin. This reaction, converting a free amino group to an amide, also converts the group from being a strong base to being neutral. The nitrogen is no longer ionizable, and is therefore no longer a barrier to the molecule's being able to cross membranes.

The next step in the sequence, catalyzed by 5-hydroxy indole-O-methyl transferase (5-HIOMT), converts the hydroxyl to a methoxy group, thereby rendering it more neutral as well. As a result of these two modifications, the melatonin molecule is now neutral and hydrophobic, whereas serotonin is basic and hydrophilic. Serotonin does not easily cross membranes, whereas melatonin is much more likely to do so.

Characteristics of Melatonin

Melatonin is a hormone with many of the characteristics of steroid hormones, because of its hydrophobic properties and the fact that it crosses membranes readily. Melatonin receptors that, like steroid hormone receptors, are soluble proteins that bind the hormone in the cytoplasm of the cell, have been identified. Receptor binding allows the complex to interact with other parts of the cell, including the genome. Therefore, melatonin, like steroid hormones, can change the level of expression of gene products by interacting with the genes directly. Such a mechanism allows the hormone to produce longer-lasting effects, since changes of genomic expression can produce effects that last for months.

Melatonin is known to produce long-term effects, including setting the yearly time for mating in some mammalian species (so the young are born in the spring) and increasing body heat production during the colder months. Other chemical products of the pineal gland, also made from serotonin, have melatonin-like hormonal effects. These are reduced and methylated forms of serotonin, 5-hydroxy tryptophol and 5-methoxy tryptophol (Figure 7-2).

The pineal body, sometimes more romantically known as the "third eye," is responsive to and regulated by ambient light. In species up to and including birds, the pineal body is directly light responsive (even through the skull and feathers). In higher animals, it is controlled indirectly by light falling on the eyes. A lengthy nerve pathway connects the visual system with the pineal body, via the hypothalamus and the brain stem. This pathway, at its terminus on the pineal body, is noradrenergic.

During darkness, noradrenaline release is elevated. Light falling on the animal's eyes inhibits this release. In the dark, NE activates the beta (and some alpha) receptors on pineal cells (pinealocytes), which in turn stimulates adenylyl cyclase and increases cyclic AMP in the pinealocytes. This, in turn, stimulates the phosphorylation of the N-acetyl transferase (NAT), the rate-limiting enzyme of melatonin synthesis. The phosphorylated form of NAT is more active, and therefore melatonin production in the pineal body is high during darkness. Melatonin inhibits sexual activity by gonad inhibition. This inhibition apparently is heightened during the early winter when periods of darkness are increasing. In the early spring, when periods of daylight increase in duration, the nerve pathway to the pineal body inhibits the release of noradrenaline onto pinealocytes, thereby decreasing production of melatonin and increasing sexual activity.

Different species respond to this effect at different times, ranging from midwinter, when days first lengthen, to later in the spring. For many mammals, this mechanism appears to be the determining factor by which light controls the timing of mating. In this way, newborns have the opportunity to experience the summer season first, undergoing winter only later, after having grown and gained strength.

Besides this effect on sexual activity, melatonin also regulates thermogenesis of brown adipose tissue (BAT). This organ, found within all fat deposits, burns metabolic fuel solely for the production of heat. This is done in such a way that ATP is not produced. Therefore, the resultant metabolic energy cannot be used for any biochemical or physiological work. In human adults, BAT is concentrated between the scapulae, on the back of the neck, and along the main blood vessels of the abdomen, in addition to its apparent universal dispersion within white adipose tissue. BAT is now known to be present in human adults, although it was long believed to be found only in infants.

BAT cells have special mitochondria that contain a protein called thermogenin, or uncoupler protein (UCP). UCP uncouples mitochondrial oxidative phosphorylation from the production of ATP. UCP does this by allowing hydroxide (OH^-) ions to flow down their concentration gradient, which is out of the mitochondrial matrix and into the intermembrane space surrounding each mitochondrion. Since the intermembrane space maintains a high concentration of H^+, the resulting reaction produces water and generates a great deal of heat and no ATP. Therefore, the addition of UCP to normally respiring mitochondria causes the production of large amounts of heat. This is the mechanism used by hibernating animals, such as bears and squirrels, to bring their bodies back to a normal temperature prior to leaving hibernation each spring. Other animals, such as humans, use this mechanism each winter as an aid in maintaining body temperature.

Although melatonin is not required for thermogenesis by BAT, it has a **trophic** effect on BAT, stimulating **hypertrophy** of the tissue by an unknown mechanism. By increasing the number of BAT cells (i.e., adipose cells that contain thermogenin), melatonin increases the amount of heat the organism is capable of producing from BAT. The BAT NE receptor is a type of beta receptor and appears to be distinct from other beta receptors. The designation β-3 has been proposed for it. There is considerable interest in this receptor in the pharmaceutical industry, since β-3 agonist drugs could theoretically be used to reduce body weight by increasing heat production. One obvious danger to this approach is cross reactivity by the drugs with other beta receptors. Such cross reactions could, for example, affect the function of the heart.

Depression

Both serotonin and melatonin have been linked to depression in some people. Serotonin has been linked directly, as mentioned above. People who die by suicide have been reported to have increased levels of serotonin in their brain stems at autopsy, and 5-HIAA levels are higher in some patients during depression.

Melatonin has been linked indirectly to depression, primarily to the depressed state some people experience during long, dark winters. Near the Arctic Circle, from Alaska to Scandinavia, many people have been reported to experience a particular kind of midwinter depression called seasonal affective disorder (SAD). Some of these patients respond to phototherapy, i.e., being placed in artificially high ambient light conditions.

SELF-STUDY QUESTIONS

Facts:

1. What effects does serotonin have on the organism?

2. What effects does serotonin have on an organism's postsynaptic cells?

Concepts:

1. Explain the mechanism by which insulin affects the synthesis of serotonin in the CNS.

2. Explain the use of CSF levels of 5-HIAA to determine possible serotonin involvement in psychiatric diseases.

3. Explain the regulation of the pineal body's production of melatonin and related hormonal products.

4. Discuss the possible mechanisms of drug-induced hallucinations via interaction with the serotonergic system.

5. Discuss the basis of phototherapy for seasonal affective disorder.

6. Describe the relationship between mating in lower mammals and melatonin levels.

BIBLIOGRAPHY

Frazer, A., Saul, M., and Wolfe, B.B. 1990. Subtypes of receptors for serotonin. *Annual Review of Pharmacology* 30: 307–348.

Julius, D. 1991. Molecular biology of serotonin receptors. *Annual Review of Neuroscience* 14: 335–360.

CHAPTER 8

Peptide Neurotransmitters

For many years peptides have been known to exist within the CNS, but an awareness of the large number of peptides that serve as neurotransmitters is relatively recent. The discovery in 1975 of the enkephalins and their role as endogenous ligands for opiate receptors initiated an explosion of neuropeptide research that continues to the present. It is now generally acknowledged that peptide transmitters exist throughout the CNS. In some parts of the brain, most notably the hypothalamus, peptides are believed to account for the bulk of transmitter activity. Therefore, peptide neurotransmitters have varied functions, and are involved in most CNS activities. A few useful generalizations can be made, however.

Within the hypothalamus, and in the axon terminals arising from hypothalamic neurons, peptides are probably the most common transmitters. In most of these tracts, the peptides function in a manner similar to the second level transmitters discussed in Chapter 3: many of the peptide-containing pathways of hypothalamic origin are associated with specific neural functions. For example, CCK-8 (see below) in the ventro-medial nucleus of the hypothalamus (VMH) appears to have a role in determining the cessation of eating. Outside the hypothalamus, many peptides function in more restricted ways, often as modulators of the synapses of other transmitters. There are **peptidergic** synapses outside the hypothalamus, however, in which the peptide is associated with particular functions as well. For example, there is a pathway near the **midbrain** in which angiotensin II is the transmitter. This tract may be part of a system for determining thirst, as the injection of angiotensin II into the tract causes experimental animals to drink water.

The enkephalins constitute one of the largest classes of peptide transmitters. They are frequently found in presynaptic synapses. Such **axo-axonic** connections often use physiological mechanisms that are distinct from those used by the more commonly considered axo-somatic and axo-dendritic synapses. Axo-axonic synapses may, in fact, be thought of as a separate category of transmitter function. The ionic mechanisms for presynaptic inhibition, for example, are significantly different from the most common postsynaptic hyperpolarizing mechanisms, such as GABA's Cl^- channel receptors discussed earlier.

An early concept of peptide transmitters, called the "gut–brain axis," led investigators to the discovery of several brain peptides. It may not have correctly explained their functions, however. The original concept proposed that many gut peptide hormones were also present in brain, sometimes in a modified form, and that a molecule's function in the two organs was similar in terms of its effects on the organism. For example, cholecystokinin (CCK) is a gut hormone involved in gall bladder emptying, and it is also found in the VMH, where it has a role in **satiety** (inhibiting further eating). After the discovery of many neuropeptides, however, the gut–brain concept no longer appeared to be compelling. Its main value, in retrospect, may have been the stimulation of the search for gut peptides in brain. Essentially, all of those that were sought were found in the CNS.

Besides the hypothalamic peptides, those found in specific tracts within the brain, and those found at presynaptic sites, there is yet another group of neuropeptides. The functions of this last group are unaccounted for, although their presence implies function. For example, unusually large quantities of CCK-8, as well as another gut peptide, VIP (vasoactive intestinal peptide), are found in neurons in the cerebral cortex, and they have no well-defined function. The majority of different kinds of transmitters within the CNS are peptides, and they most likely play some role in nearly all brain functions.

PEPTIDE SYNTHESIS

Much of the current research on neuropeptides is focused on the gene products from which they are made, on their mechanism of action at synapses, and on the elucidation of the physiological functions they determine. All known peptide neurotransmitters are synthesized on ribosomes as portions of precursor proteins (which are the actual gene products). None of the peptide neurotransmitters are known to be synthesized by direct, specific enzyme action using free amino acids (as is **glutathione,** for example). Five gene products from which neurotransmitter peptides are made have been well characterized, and enough is known about them and their peptide transmitter derivatives to form a few generalizations.

Genes that encode proteins often encode sequences of amino acids that do not appear in the final products. These larger precursors are called **proproteins** (for example, proenkephalins; see below). An additional sequence, usually near the N terminus, serves as a "signal" for crossing membranes. Precursor proteins that contain this signal peptide, in addition to other sequences that will be trimmed out later, are called **preproproteins.** Many precursors for neuropeptides contain sequences that appear to be such signal regions.

The ways in which genes are processed to produce protein products is highly complex in the CNS, with the same gene being able to produce different protein or peptide products in different cells. The sources of this heterogeneity appear to be both at the messenger RNA level and at the level of the protein itself. At the moment, the mechanisms used by different neurons to produce different proteins from the same gene are not entirely known. There is evidence to indicate that both **post-transcriptional** mechanisms (i.e., modifications of the messenger RNA) and **post-translational** mechanisms (i.e., modifications of the protein after it is synthesized) are used.

Neuropeptide protein precursors may contain multiple copies of the active peptides. The total number of active products from each precursor protein, however, is small. Protachykinin, for example, has a single copy each of substance P and of substance K; see Table 8-1. **Proopiomelanocortin (POMC),** the precursor protein for beta endorphin in the arcuate nuclei of the hypothalamus, contains only a single copy of active endorphin, in addition to single copies of adrenocorticotrophic hormone (ACTH) and gamma melanocyte–stimulating hormone. Each of these precursors has multiple active peptides, but only one copy of a particular neuropeptide.

Since neuropeptide precursors are made ribosomally, and protein synthesis does not occur in axons or terminals, they must be synthesized in the cell body and subsequently transported to the synaptic terminal. Along the way, the hydrolytic processing necessary to produce active peptides occurs in the transport vesicles.

A large part of this preparative hydrolysis is accomplished by trypsin-like proteases, which specifically cleave the precursors at sites where basic amino acids occur in tandem (Figure 8-1). Most active neuropeptides exist within their precursors surrounded by such pairs of the basic amino acids, e.g., arginine **(R)** and lysine **(K).**

In addition to being freed from their precursors by hydrolysis, many peptides require further enzymatic modification before becoming active. All neuropeptides would have a positively charged amino group at one end and a negatively charged carboxyl group at the other if they were simply freed by hydrolysis from the parent protein. The most common neuropeptide modifications are changes in these charged groups, creating neutral amides at one or both ends of the peptide. Such modifications remove the charges from the terminal groups, and generate structures that are reasonably chemically stable. The advantage of such modifications to the transmitters appears to be in making them resistant to hydrolysis once they are released from the cell into the extracellular fluid of the synaptic cleft. (Most CNS extracellular **peptidases** require either a free, positively charged amino terminal or a free, negatively charged carboxyl terminal in order to be active.)

The most common neutralizations of the charges are the formation of a simple amide at the C terminal and acetylation of the N terminal. An acetyl group is transferred from an acetyl CoA to the N terminus of the peptide after its release from its precursor. Amidation of the C terminal is often accomplished by the action of a special enzyme, **peptidyl glycine alpha-amidating monooxygenase (PAM).** This process requires oxygen, vitamin C, and Cu^{++} as cofactors. PAM's action requires that the peptide be released from its precursor with a glycine residue attached to its C-terminal amino acid. The enzyme is actually an oxidase that oxidizes and releases the two carbons of the glycine as carbon dioxide, leaving the glycine's nitrogen atom as an amide. This action results in a neutral C terminal on the peptide (Figure 8-2).

Figure 8-1 General Structure of a Preproprotein (Gene Product)

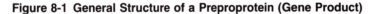
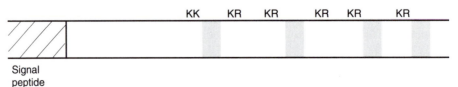

Signal
peptide

Table 8-1 A Sampling of Important Neuropeptides

Precursor	Peptide	Structure[1]
Procholecystokinin	CCK-8	DY (SO$_3$$^-$) MGWMDF-NH$_2$[2]
Protachykinin	Substance P	RPKPQQFFGLM-NH$_2$
	Substance K	HKTDS FVGLM-NH$_2$
Proenkephalin A	MENK	YGGFM
	LENK	YGGFL
	Heptapeptide	YGGFMRF
	Octapeptide	YGGFMRGL
	Peptide E	YGGFMRRVGRPEWWMDYQKRYGGFL
Proenkephalin B (prodynorphin)	LENK	YGGFL
	Alpha neoendorphin	YGGFLRKYPK
	Beta neoendorphin	YGGFLRKYP
	Dynorphin A (1–17)	YGGFLRRIRPKLKWDNQ
	Dynorphin B (1–8)	YGGFLRRI
	Leumorphin (dynorphin B) (1–29)	YGGFLRRQFKVVTRSQQDPNAYYEELFDV
	Dynorphin B (rimorphin)	YGGFLRRQFKVVT
Propiomelanocortin (POMC)	Beta endorphin	YGGFLTSEKSQTPLVTLFKNAIIKNAYKKGE
	Adrenocorticotrophic hormone (ACTH)	SYSMEHFRWGKPVGKKRRPVKVYPDAGEDQSAEAFPLEF
Other	Angiotensin II	DRVYIHPF
	Bradykinin	RPPGFSPFR
	Vasoactive intestinal peptide (VIP)	HSDAVFTDNYTRLRKEMAVKKYLNSILN-NH$_2$
	Corticotropin-releasing hormone (CRF)	SEEPPISLDLTFHLLREVLEMARAQQLAQQAHSNRKLMEII-NH$_2$

[1]Standard abbreviations: (A) alanine, (C) cysteine, (D) aspartate, (E) glutamate, (F) phenylalanine, (G) glycine, (H) histidine, (I) isoleucine, (K) lysine, (L) leucine, (M) methionine, (N) asparagine, (P) proline, (Q) glutamine, (R) arginine, (S) serine, (T) threonine, (V) valine, (W) tryptophan, (Y) tyrosine
[2]All structures are written with the N terminal on the left and the C terminal on the right, as is the convention. -NH$_2$ at the C terminal means that it carries an amide group and is therefore neutral. The word "acetyl" at the N terminal indicates that the terminal amino group is acetylated and is therefore neutral. Without any such special indication, the N and C termini are assumed to be free and charged.

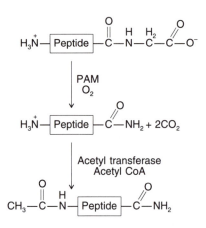

**Figure 8-2 Amidation
of Peptides for
Protection from
Peptidases**

Substance P (Table 8-1), for example, containing twelve amino acids, is released from its precursor protein with a C-terminal sequence of methioninyl-glycine. The two carbons of the glycine residue are then oxidized as described above, leaving an amide group on the now C-terminal methionine residue of a peptide containing only eleven amino acids. This is the active form of substance P.

An example of another type of post-translational modification that is necessary to make an active neuropeptide is the sulfation of CCK-8. The active peptide contains a sulfate residue in ester linkage on the side chain of a tyrosine. The peptide is inactive in vivo without the sulfate group.

The enzymatic processes that form the active neuropeptides take place both in the neuronal perikarya and in the axon while the peptide is being transported to its site of storage in the terminal. Once a peptide is released from the cell that synthesized it, it produces its characteristic postsynaptic action, and apparently is then promptly hydrolyzed to inactive amino acids and smaller peptides by the extracellular peptidases of the synaptic cleft.

NEUROPEPTIDE PRECURSORS

There are at least five well-characterized neuropeptide precursors: procholecystokinin, protachykinin, and three proenkephalins (propiomelanocortin, proenkephalin A, and proenkephalin B). Each is discussed separately below.

Procholecystokinin

Procholecystokinin is a peptide precursor found in both the cerebral cortex and the hypothalamus. Its only known products are cholecystokinins, the best-characterized of which range in size from four to thirty-three amino acids. Each precursor molecule may contain only one active peptide, however.

As mentioned above, the protein product of a single gene may be different in different neurons. There is heterogeneity among the neuropeptide products as well. CCK illustrates this point well, as there are multiple active forms of CCK. Cholecystokinin, as a gut hormone, has thirty-three amino acids. Most attention in the CNS has been focused on CCK-8, which contains the eight C-terminal amino acids of the larger molecule. CCK-4, having only four C-terminal amino acids, is also found in significant quantity. The degree of neuropeptide activity of the largest and the smallest forms is not known, but this kind of neuropeptide heterogeneity of structure is common. (This point will be made more strongly in a later discussion of the enkephalin family.)

The function of hypothalamic CCK-8 has been mentioned; the role of the comparatively large amounts of CCK-8 in the cerebral cortex is yet unknown.

Protachykinin

Protachykinin is the name given the precursor for substance P and substance K. The gene for these peptides can be processed in different ways in different cells. As a result, some cells produce only substance P. In others, each precursor contains a copy of each of the two peptides. Substance K, previously known as a peptide in amphibians, was discovered in brain by determining the structure of protachykinin. A receptor for substance K has also been found in brain, but its function is still not characterized. This peptide is now often referred to as neuromedin A.

Substance P, the first neuropeptide discovered, is known to be the transmitter for primary **sensory afferents,** in addition to being a transmitter for tracts in higher parts of the brain. Therefore, it is the main transmitter by which pain signals are transmitted from the periphery to higher brain centers. In some locations, such as tooth pulp, all neurons that send axons to other regions use substance P as their transmitter. Such centers are specialized for the transmission of pain, but they also contain presynaptic synapses that can modulate the transmission of the pain signal. These presynaptic synapses are also peptidergic, and often are enkephalinergic (see below).

Proenkephalins

There are three well-characterized precursors that contain neuropeptides related to enkephalins. The combination of all three gene products provides a large number of peptides that have enkephalin-like functions. These different classes of peptides, with possibly similar functions, have been given several different names: enkephalins, endorphins, dynorphins, rimorphins, etc. All refer to molecules that can be grouped into one large class (neuropeptides that bind to morphine receptors) which is subdivided into three or more smaller classes based on the molecules' proproteins.

Proopiomelanocortin (POMC) was one of the first precursors to be **sequenced.** One precursor molecule yields one molecule of active beta endorphin, one molecule of adrenocorticotrophic hormone (ACTH), and one molecule of gamma melanocyte–stimulating hormone (MSH). Beta endorphin is a C-terminal extension of leu-enkephalin (LENK) containing a total of thirty-one amino acid residues. The gamma MSH may be an inactive form of the hormone. At first it was thought that POMC might always produce ACTH and beta endorphin in a one-to-one ratio. This was especially thought to be the case in the pituitary gland, in which large amounts of POMC can be found. A more current view holds that precursor proteins can be processed in different ways in different cells.

Proenkephalin A, first discovered in adrenal medulla, is also synthesized in the CNS. Each precursor molecule may contain both forms of enkephalin, met-enkephalin (MENK) and leu-enkephalin (LENK), usually in a ratio of 4:1. It may also contain other peptides related to these, most of which are extensions of MENK at its C terminal. MENK and LENK have similar efficacy at many receptors. This may be due to the fact that their only structural difference is the C-terminal amino acid.

Proenkephalin B, sometimes called prodynorphin, contains LENK in addition to molecules called dynorphins, rimorphins, and neoendorphins. All of these are C-terminal extensions of LENK; up to twenty-four amino acids are present in the extension, beyond the five present in LENK.

All the peptides from proenkephalins A and B, as well as beta endorphin and some of its smaller derivatives, are able to act upon enkephalin receptors. In fact, the most active ligands for some of these receptors may be the longer forms.

PEPTIDE CATABOLISM

One of the more puzzling aspects of neuropeptide function is their apparent hydrolysis to component amino acids and peptides in the synaptic cleft. Experimental data indicate that hydrolysis is the method of synaptic inactivation, and that it occurs quite rapidly. This places neuropeptides in a class with acetylcholine as being transmitters that are inactivated by hydrolysis after use, rather than being recycled.

In the case of neuropeptides, such a situation appears to be much more wasteful of energy and substrates than it is in the case of acetylcholine, since peptides cannot be resynthesized at the synaptic terminal. There are no ribosomes in axons or their terminals and, therefore, protein synthesis in these locations is not possible. The hydrolysis of peptides after their release is the culmination of several energy-demanding processes that begin with the synthesis of the precursor protein in the perikaryon and continue during transport to the terminal. This journey requires several minutes to an hour or more, depending on the length of the axon. Ultimately, peptide hydrolysis may culminate outside the cell, in the synaptic cleft, with complete hydrolysis to individual amino acids. Without the recycling of peptides, replenishing the supply of transmitter at the terminal requires new perikaryal synthesis and transport. This appears to be a highly energy inefficient system.

An additional problem is the loss of rapid homeostasis. If the amount of peptide transmitter were acutely depleted at a terminal, a significant delay prior to replenishment of adequate stores might ensue. At present, the evolutionary utility of this system is not clear.

Two classes of extracellular synaptic peptidases are most prominent: carboxypeptidases and aminopeptidases. Both of these are further subdivided. Carboxypeptidases require their substrate to have a charged carboxyl group at the C terminal. The enzyme then hydrolyzes the peptide bond for which it is specific. The earliest-known carboxypeptidases hydrolyze the peptide bond closest to the C terminal, i.e., the bond that joins the last two amino acids to each other. In addition to this type of carboxypeptidase, the synaptic clefts of the CNS also contain carboxypeptidases specific for the second peptide bond from the C-terminal

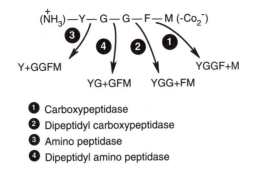

- ❶ Carboxypeptidase
- ❷ Dipeptidyl carboxypeptidase
- ❸ Amino peptidase
- ❹ Dipeptidyl amino peptidase

Figure 8-3 The Extracellular Hydrolysis of Neuropeptides

residue, i.e., that between the second and third amino acids from the end. Since one product of this reaction is a dipeptide (i.e., two amino acids joined by a peptide bond), these enzymes are called dipeptidyl carboxypeptidases. Reactions 1 and 2 in Figure 8-3 illustrate the actions of these two types of carboxypeptidase.

There are other enzymes with analogous specificities for hydrolysis of peptides at the other end, the N terminus. Aminopeptidases specifically cleave the peptide bond closest to the N terminus, and dipeptidyl amino peptidases yield a dipeptide as one product (steps 3 and 4 in Figure 8-3). In tests of enkephalins in vivo, the major cleavage of the peptide is by a dipeptidyl carboxypeptidase and the secondary cleavage is by a traditional aminopeptidase. The former enzyme is sometimes referred to as "enkephalinase." As discussed above, modifications of neuropeptides that remove the charge on either terminal group make the peptide resistant to hydrolysis by these enzymes. The most common of such modifications, the addition of acetyl groups on the N terminus and amide groups on the C terminus, achieve this purpose. With either group, the resulting peptide has a longer active life between its release from its terminal and when it is destroyed. Although these peptides are probably not recycled, as some other transmitters are, they do have a prolonged effect. In the case of enkephalins, neither the C-terminal nor the N-terminal group is modified in vivo. The C-terminal negative charge can be removed without affecting activity, however. The N-terminal tyrosine must have a positive charge, or the peptide is inactive.

NEUROPEPTIDE SYNAPSES

The enkephalinergic synapses have been studied in great detail. Although widely spread throughout the CNS, they are frequently found in presynaptic, axo-axonic locations. Here, enkephalins affect other synaptic terminals, changing the release of the second transmitter. This, of course, means they have only an indirect effect on the major postsynaptic cell. The general effect of enkephalins is inhibitory, resulting in a decreased release of transmitter from the presynaptic terminals they modulate. The neurophysiological mechanism of this effect is somewhat different from that of inhibitory postsynaptic receptors, although it also involves an increase in K^+ conductance.

Increasing K^+ permeability in a presynaptic terminal causes a decrease in subsequent presynaptic potentials, in the following way. Since the later part, or the recovery portion, of a membrane potential is produced by K^+ ions flowing back into the terminal, increasing this permeability diminishes the total time required for a potential (see Figure 3-2, page 35). This diminution results in a lowered Ca^{++} mobilization at the terminal and, therefore, in a decreased release of transmitter from the terminal's storage vesicles. These postsynaptic effects of enkephalins (on the presynaptic terminal of another transmitter) are sometimes associated with decreased levels of cAMP. An example of this kind of arrangement is in tooth pulp, mentioned above as containing substance P neurons. These neurons' terminals have enkephalinergic synapses on them, and increasing the release of enkephalins decreases the amount of substance P released, thereby decreasing the perception of pain from the tooth. In fact, this mechanism has been purported to be a part of the placebo effect for anesthesia. An innocuous drug (i.e., a placebo) believed by the patient to be an anesthetic can apparently diminish the release of substance P through the enkephalinergic effect in about 40 percent of patients. A powerful inhibitor of enkephalinergic receptors, naloxone, has been shown to prevent such a placebo effect in subjects undergoing root canal procedures.

Enkephalin synapses, as well as those of other peptides, often have different kinetic properties from those of other kinds of transmitters. Peptide synapses tend to fire in bursts, for example. Continuous release of peptide may produce no measurable effect, but releasing the same peptide, in the same pathway, at a rate of one synaptic release per hour may produce the effect. This type of synaptic behavior may be a part of the explanation for the point made earlier, that it takes a comparatively long time to restore peptides to a terminal once they have been depleted.

ENKEPHALIN RECEPTORS

The receptors for the enkephalin class of transmitters have been studied intensely for many years. Opiate drugs interact with some of the same receptors, so there is considerable interest in attempting to develop drugs that have some opiate properties (e.g., analgesia) without being as subject to abuse and as likely to lead to addiction as the opiates that are currently used clinically.

Current research has identified three classes of opiate receptors: mu, delta, and kappa. All are bound by the highly potent opiate antagonist naloxone. Because naloxone binds strongly to opiate receptors and displaces agonists, acute administration of naloxone is able to precipitate an opiate withdrawal syndrome in an addict.

A fourth class of enkephalin receptor, the sigma receptor, has been described. This receptor does not bind naloxone, however. Therefore, strictly speaking, it is not an opiate receptor, by current definition. All endogenous opiates (enkephalins, dynorphins, rymorphins, beta-endorphin, etc.) have some ability to bind all three major classes of receptor. Each has specificity for one or more classes, however.

Mu Receptor

Mu receptors (Greek μ, for morphine) have been studied longest. One of their interesting properties is that the binding of enkephalins to mu receptors is strongly influenced by Na^+ ion concentration. The higher the Na^+ concentration, the lower the binding affinity (and the better antagonists are bound). Evidence gathered from early attempts to isolate mu receptors also indicates that sulfatides may be involved in their stereospecific binding. Therefore, sulfatides may be present in or bound to the mu receptor. (This point is not widely accepted, however.) Heroin, morphine, and most other opiates that are subject to abuse either serve as or are converted to powerful agonists for mu receptors. Indeed, even many of the side effects of heroin usage, such as constipation, can be explained by its agonist properties for mu receptors everywhere in the body. The gastrointestinal tract, as well as the CNS, has mu receptors.

CNS mu receptors are in highest concentration in the thalamus, hypothalamus, hippocampus, and periaqueductal gray. All of these structures are known also to contain high concentrations of one or more endogenous opioid peptides.

Delta Receptors

Delta receptors are named for the Greek letter delta, which is used to identify the vas deferens, from which these receptors were first isolated. Delta receptors are concentrated in the CNS in the amygdala and nucleus accumbens. Enkephalins appear to be most highly associated with delta receptors in vivo, and thus may be their major physiological agonist.

Kappa Receptors

Kappa receptors, the function of which is probably the least well known, are found in greatest abundance in the deep cortex, cerebellum, hypothalamus, neostriatum, and spinal cord. They appear to work by decreasing Ca^{++} permeability and, therefore, probably act by hyperpolarizing or inhibiting receptors on a postsynaptic cell. The name of this class comes from the name of a drug (ketocyclazocine) used experimentally for its preferential binding to kappa receptors. In vivo, dynorphins may be the preferential ligands for kappa receptors.

SELF-STUDY QUESTIONS

Facts:

1. What are the structures of MENK and LENK?

2. Which intracellular enzymes are necessary to convert the precursor proteins into active neuropeptides?

3. What kinds of messenger RNAs have been characterized for neuropeptides?

4. Describe one role and location for each of the following: substance P, CCK-8, MENK.

5. Describe the modifications that occur to peptide terminals in order to increase their synaptic life.

6. Describe the enzymes that degrade neuropeptides in their synapses.

Concepts:

1. Describe the mechanism by which MENK decreases the release of substance P in a pain pathway.

2. Describe the time frame for the action of peptides.

3. Discuss the gut-brain axis hypothesis.

BIBLIOGRAPHY

Brownstein, M. 1989. Neuropeptides. In *Basic Neurochemistry*, edited by G. Siegel, B. Agranoff, R.W. Albers, and P. Molinoff. New York: Raven Press.

Lynch, D., and Snyder, S. 1986. Neuropeptides: Multiple molecular forms, metabolic pathways, and receptors. *Annual Review of Biochemistry* 55: 773–799.

Simon, E.J., and Miller, J.M. 1989. Opioid peptides and opioid receptors. In *Basic Neurochemistry*, edited by G. Siegel, B. Agranoff, R.W. Albers, and P. Molinoff. New York: Raven Press.

Receptors

CHAPTER 9

Neurotransmitter Direct Receptors

During the initial phase of neurotransmitter discovery, there was often a focus on relating specific transmitters to specific neural functions. This type of correlation can be made in some cases, but the total picture is now known to be more complicated. Several dozen transmitters are currently known, each of which utilizes multiple receptors. In order to understand the correlations between molecular changes within the brain and a particular mental function, one must have knowledge of multiple factors, not just knowledge of the particular transmitter. The nature of the receptor(s) involved is one of the most important of these factors.

RECEPTOR CATEGORIES

There are two distinct categories of neurotransmitter receptors, those that are ion channels and those that involve some type of "second messenger" system, and each category has several subtypes. Each of these categories has several names. Ion channels are frequently called "ionotropic" or "ligand-activated" receptors. Those that use second messengers are often referred to as "metabotropic" or "second messenger" receptors. Here the types will be called "direct" and "indirect" receptors (see Chapter 11), respectively. By definition, all receptors contain the molecules or subunits that actually bind the transmitter. Most receptors, of either type, have in common the fact that they are located within the membrane, thus spanning it, but also having portions of their molecule(s) in both the intra- and the extracellular aqueous compartments.

Direct receptors are macromolecular complexes that comprise an ion channel and its regulatory mechanism. Many have now been cloned and sequenced. They are structurally and mechanistically analogous to allosteric enzymes. These channel complexes are composed of multiple polypeptide chains that are associated with each other by non-covalent forces and are contained within the hydrophobic region of the cells' plasma membranes. Each protein subunit contains multiple transmembrane segments (often four), and each transmembrane segment is an alpha helix. Despite the fact that these helices are in a hydrophobic environment, they are excellent examples of the classical protein helical structure predicted in the 1950s by Linus Pauling. Each transmembrane helix typically consists of about twenty to twenty-three amino acids.

Together, the multiple subunits of the ion channel form an allosteric complex. The complex is activated by the binding of the appropriate transmitter (Figure 9-1). Typically, these receptors require two or more molecules of the transmitter to be bound simultaneously in order to open the channel. This requirement arises from the channel's containing two or more copies of the polypeptide subunit that bears the transmitter binding site. Figure 9-1 shows one version of the GABA-A receptor, the most common postsynaptic receptor for GABA. The figure depicts only two kinds of subunits (alpha and beta) and two copies of each. The binding sites for GABA were initially thought to be associated with the alpha subunits, implying that two GABA molecules were required. The modern view of this receptor, however, is much more complex: it is now thought to contain as many as seven subunits of five different kinds. The receptor can function with only the four subunits it was earlier thought to contain, however. When the information for only those four proteins was injected into *Xenopus laevis* **oocytes,** apparently functional receptors were made by the oocytes, and expressed in their membranes. This may be the simplest fully functional example of a direct receptor, although it is a research form and not the one found in vivo.

When the correct number and type of transmitter molecules bind to appropriate sites, a conformational change occurs among the subunits, resulting in the opening of the ion channel. The channel is a pore through the membrane, which is selective for one or more ions of a particular charge. In the best-known cases, involving the nicotinic acetyl choline and the GABA-A receptors, the channel is centrally located within the complex. Each of the major protein subunits contributes a portion of the channel (helix 2 in Figure 9-1). Each subunit thus contributes one or more of its helices to create an aqueous compartment within the membrane. The remaining transmembrane helices in each subunit are entirely surrounded by the hydrophobic lipid membrane (Figure 9-1). Therefore, protein subunits of this receptor class have one or more alpha helices that must contain some hydrophilic amino acid side chains, as these side chains must be able to

Figure 9-1 Model of the topology of the GABA-A receptor alpha and beta subunits. *Putative membrane-spanning helices are depicted as cylinders. Potential sites for N-glycosylation are indicated by triangles. A consensus site for serine phosphorylation by protein kinase A, which is present only in the beta subunit, is indicated by a circled P.*

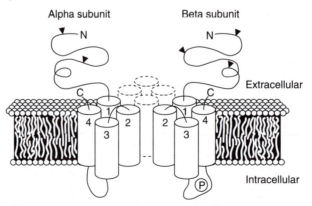

interact with water molecules when the channel is open. In fact, hydrophilic residues occur in approximately every third position in one of the alpha helices of each subunit.

In addition to the transmitter binding sites and the helices that make up the channel, a direct receptor may have additional special features. Some of these are part of the regulatory systems for opening the channel. Other special features may determine the specificity for the ions allowed to pass through the channel. For example, the GABA-A receptor is a chloride channel, and therefore, in addition to its regulatory mechanisms, the receptor complex must contain a "selectivity filter" that chooses Cl^- over other ions.

Subtypes of Direct Receptors

The two most general categories of all receptors are excitatory (i.e., producing epsp's) and inhibitory (producing ipsp's). Each of these classes has several subdivisions, based on the kinds of ligands required to activate the receptor complex, the kind(s) of ions whose permeability is affected, and whether ion permeability is increased or decreased. Since the normal charge across a neuron's membrane is negative on the cytoplasmic side, any permeability change that increases negative charges in the cytoplasm is hyperpolarizing, or inhibitory, and any change that decreases this voltage is depolarizing, or excitatory.

In this context, increases of Na^+ ion permeability are excitatory, because the sodium flows predominantly inward and is depolarizing. Decreases of K^+ ion permeability are also excitatory, and increases are inhibitory. This latter situation results from potassium's being high inside the cell, and an increase in its permeability causes an outward flow. Increases of Cl^- ion permeability are inhibitory, at least in part because of a resulting hyperpolarization, and decreases in Na^+ ion permeability are also inhibitory.

DIRECT RECEPTOR REGULATION

Each receptor complex has multiple levels of regulation, analogous to those for allosteric enzymes. Short-term regulation (milliseconds) is allosteric and controlled by binding transmitter and other regulatory molecules. Covalent modifications require a longer time to take effect and also last longer (i.e., from hundreds of milliseconds to seconds). Covalent modifications may override allosteric effects. The most common covalent regulation is reversible protein phosphorylation–dephosphorylation.

Over a longer time span (minutes to hours or longer), regulation of the number of receptor molecules in a given cell occurs. Regulation can occur from modifications in the rate of either synthesis or catabolism. Changes in synthesis can occur at the level of either **transcription** or **translation.** Of these longer-term regulations of receptor number, the fastest are likely due to increased catabolism; changes of synthesis take place over the longest period.

In the time span of a single synaptic event, at least two of these levels of regulation may be operative. Transmitter release allosterically opens the receptor's ionophore (the ion channel), and the receptor may be inactivated by a phosphorylation shortly thereafter. In this case, as in many others, phosphorylation serves as an override mechanism for the short-term allosteric control.

The addition of one or more phosphates to the receptor is possibly a timing mechanism designed to prevent the allosteric effects from lasting too long. (Examples of other such timing mechanisms are discussed in Chapters 10 and 11 with regard to **G proteins,** where the slowness of the enzymatic action of the G protein is also such a timing device.) In fact, many receptors of both direct and indirect types may have a protein kinase physically associated with them, more or less as one of the subunits. This kinase, when activated, adds a phosphate group from ATP to one or more amino acid side chains on the protein subunits that constitute the channel. This phosphorylation markedly changes the conformation (and therefore the allosteric properties) of the protein.

Conformational States of the Receptor

In the direct receptors that have been most extensively studied to date, this combination of allosteric and phosphorylation regulation produces at least three separate states of the receptor. These have been called, in the case of the nicotinic receptor for acetylcholine, the "resting (R)," "active (A)," and "desensitized (D)" states. In the R state, the channel is closed, and the receptor's K_D (i.e., binding affinity) for the transmitter is intermediate. In the A state, the channel is open, and the K_D for transmitter is high (that is, the transmitter does not bind well). In the D state, the channel is closed, but the K_D for transmitter is typically low (that is, the transmitter binds well or may still be tightly bound) (Figure 9-2). The D state is

Figure 9-2 Three States of an Ion Channel Receptor

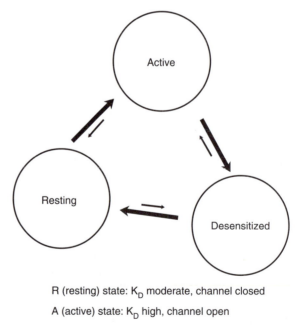

R (resting) state: K_D moderate, channel closed

A (active) state: K_D high, channel open

D (desensitized) state: K_D low, channel closed

thought to be phosphorylated and, therefore, to contain a covalent override of the transmitter's signal, closing the channel regardless of the presence of transmitter.

Although it is not entirely clear, it is possible that these three states occur in sequence. Transmitter molecules bind to the R state, moving the channel to the A state. In this condition, the channel is open. A short time later, the receptor kinase converts the A to the D state, in which the channel is closed, regardless of the presence of transmitter. If this sequence does occur, there must also be a phosphatase (i.e., an enzyme to remove the phosphate groups) that converts the receptor complex back to the resting state. This, indeed, appears to be the case. There is also evidence that each of these transformations is reversible (i.e., that A can become R, D can become A, and so on).

Each state of the receptor, because it has a distinct three-dimensional structure, is susceptible to unique drug intervention. Although there are some drugs that may be able to affect all three states (e.g., alcohol), others are specific to one of the states and do not bind to the others. For example, there are drugs that specifically bind within the open ionophore of one of the acetylcholine receptors. Such a drug then blocks the channel and blocks the action of acetylcholine. Such a drug does not bind to the same site as acetylcholine itself, and therefore need not be at all similar to acetylcholine in structure. Thus, multiple receptor states give rise to multiple possible sites of intervention.

SPECIFIC DIRECT RECEPTORS

The major ligands for direct receptors in the CNS are amino acid transmitters. Amino acids are typically present in high concentrations. Each direct receptor most likely requires that two or more molecules of transmitter remain bound to it during the period of time the channel is open.

Direct receptors do not have the cascade or magnification effect observed with indirect receptors, wherein a molecule of transmitter can activate hundreds of molecules of enzyme in the postsynaptic cell (Chapters 10 and 11). Therefore, larger concentrations of transmitter are typically required for direct channels.

The inhibitory amino acids, GABA and glycine, each affect direct receptors, primarily on their postsynaptic cells. The predominant postsynaptic receptors for these two transmitters are remarkably similar to each other in overall structure and shape, although their amino acid sequences are significantly different. This illustrates greater evolutionary conservation of the **tertiary structure** of proteins than of their **primary structure.** This concept has been shown to be true for many regulated allosteric proteins, even for hemoglobin, and reinforces both the importance of protein's tertiary structure and its role in regulation, as well as the frequency of amino acid substitutions in the course of evolution.

Excitatory amino acids activate at least five different direct channels, with a variety of names, as mentioned in Chapter 4. Many of these receptors and/or their subunits have been cloned, and at least six different subunits (designated GLUR1 through GLUR6) are now known. Different excitatory amino acid receptors are most frequently designated by the names of specific artificial drug ligands, such as N-methyl-D-aspartate (NMDA), kainic acid (K), alpha-amino-3-hydroxy-5-methyl-4-isoxazoleproprionate (AMPA), etc.

GABA and Glycine Direct Receptors

GABA and glycine direct receptors are both Cl$^-$ ion channels. When the ionophore is open, chloride ions move toward equilibrium across the plasma membrane of the cell. Equilibrium is often achieved, establishing the membrane as a "chloride membrane." It is thought that the usual gradient of chloride ions is toward the cytoplasm (meaning that Cl$^-$ ions move into the cell), thus increasing the already net negative charge inside the cell and hyperpolarizing the cell's membrane.

However, even when the gradient is in the reverse direction (as occasionally occurs), the cell is still inhibited and is made more resistant to firing an action potential. As chloride ions move toward equilibrium, the postsynaptic membrane becomes stabilized by the increased ion flux across it. Thus, the stabilized cell becomes more difficult to depolarize. It is therefore inhibited from firing.

The binding sites for glycine on its postsynaptic chloride channel receptors are highly specific, both for glycine and for strychnine as an antagonist. Strychnine's well-known excitatory actions are thus attributable to its ability to block the inhibitory effect of glycine. Since glycine is the predominant inhibitory transmitter of the ventral (motor) aspect of the spinal cord, strychnine is particularly excitatory to these neurons.

A great deal of information is currently available regarding the molecular detail of the GABA-A receptor. The function of the GABA-A receptor is central to the mechanism of action of several important psychotropic drugs. For example, alcohol, barbiturates, and benzodiazepines (i.e., "tranquilizers") produce at least a part of their effects through allosteric modifications of GABA-A receptors. The specifics of these mechanisms are complex (see Chapters 13 and 17).

Benzodiazepines (BZPs) produce a tranquilizing effect and, therefore, might be expected to be GABA agonists. However, BZPs do not bind to the same binding sites or subunits as GABA molecules; therefore they have a more indirect effect. A similar situation exists for alcohol (ethanol) and many barbiturates. (Barbiturates and alcohol also have many other sites of action within the CNS and the rest of the body.)

The primary action of BZPs is their ability to enhance GABA activity at the GABA-A receptor. Although the specifics of this effect are not entirely certain, it can be described as a secondary allosteric effect. That is, BZPs, when bound to their distinct sites on separate subunits of the receptor, allosterically increase the binding of GABA to its binding sites. Additionally, GABA binds and modifies the kinetic characteristics of the complex to increase Cl$^-$ permeability. BZPs thus function as allosteric effectors of allosteric effectors. In fact, the site on the GABA-A receptor that benzodiazepines bind (and that also possibly binds ethanol and other drugs) may have an endogenous ligand. This molecule appears to be a peptide, and its normal effect is to inhibit the activity of GABA in its activation of the receptor. Therefore, this endogenous peptide produces agitation, and is sometimes called the "anxiety peptide." Benzodiazepines, ethanol, and other drugs may function as antagonists of this anxiety molecule in vivo, producing an enhancement of GABA's tranquilizing, or CNS inhibitory, effect. The regulation of the entire system is obviously mechanistically complex.

GABA also has another receptor, GABA-B, that appears to be a second messenger receptor, of the type discussed in Chapter 11.

Excitatory Amino Acid Direct Receptors

Frequently referred to as "glutamate" receptors, excitatory amino acid (EAA) receptors are probably responsive to several excitatory amino acids or their derivatives (i.e., glutamate, aspartate, N-acetyl aspartate, and possibly some small peptides containing both). The best known of these, mentioned previously, are NMDA, K, and AMPA receptors, with further subdivisions based on the actual subunit structure. There is an additional class of excitatory amino acid receptors, called metabotropic receptors, that use the second messengers **IP3** and **DAG** (Chapter 11).

When activated, direct EAA receptors are capable of causing cellular damage. This apparently can occur because it is possible to overstimulate a neuron to the point that it self-destructs. The mechanism of this effect, called "excitotoxicity," is not known in detail, but it currently is a subject of intense research.

If neurons can be overstimulated, they are capable either of overriding or bypassing the many negative feedback controls within the cell. The overstimulation results in neuronal death, possibly by self-digestion, or autolysis (the hydrolysis of some of the cell's own essential macromolecules). The fact that excitotoxicity can occur emphasizes the importance of metabolic and receptor regulation.

The agonist amino acid (e.g., glutamate) binds to all the different excitatory receptors, which are often found together in the plasma membrane of the same cell. The agonist, therefore, can produce multiple effects via a variety of receptors. There clearly is a need (both in research and in clinical practice) for drugs that bind specifically to a single type of receptor. In receptor research, it is common to designate the receptor with the initial of such a specific drug.

K Receptors

Kainic acid is one drug that binds preferentially to a single type of receptor. K receptors appear to be non-specific or "all-ion" channels. K receptors activate (depolarize) cells by allowing many positive ions through their ionophores. The flow of Na^+ ions in particular into the cell (down its gradient from the extracellular fluid) reduces the negative charge inside the cell. It thereby results in depolarization of the cell. Kainic acid has been known for some time to be lethal to neurons, especially to immature ones.

AMPA Receptors

Some AMPA receptors were first called Q receptors (for quisqualic acid) and were originally thought to be a single receptor. They have now been subdivided into at least two types, one of which is metabotropic, using second messengers. AMPA receptors are similar in function to K receptors, both being non-specific depolarizing channels. AMPA and K receptors are often found on the same neurons. Either receptor population alone can activate the neuron containing it to the point of producing an action potential.

NMDA Receptors

In recent years a major focus of research has been the NMDA (N-methyl-D-aspartate) receptor, as it appears to be the most powerful, the most complex, and possibly the most deadly of the EAA receptors. N-methyl-D-aspartate is a synthetic molecule not found in nature, which apparently binds specifically to this receptor. The NMDA receptor is unique in many ways. For example, it is the only ion channel currently known that is regulated both by a ligand (i.e., an excitatory amino acid) and by voltage. Its activation requires both a low-level depolarization (i.e., a voltage change) and the allosteric changes produced by transmitter binding.

As shown schematically in Figure 9-3, the NMDA channel in the resting state has one or more Mg^{++} ions bound in the channel on the cytoplasmic side. This Mg^{++} binding blocks the channel, thus preventing other ions from passing through. The voltage change required for NMDA receptor activation accomplishes the removal of the Mg^{++}. This voltage change is often achieved by the EAA activation of other EAA receptors, such as K or AMPA, in the same cell. In addition to this baseline depolarization, NMDA receptors require at least two allosteric ligands, the excitatory amino acid transmitter (released from a nearby cell) and glycine. Other allosteric sites are known to be part of the NMDA receptor. These include a site for Zn^{++} and another that responds to the psychotropic drug phencyclidine (PCP). The latter two sites have not been as well characterized as the others. This role of glycine in the NMDA receptor is unique. In all other known cases, glycine is an inhibitory transmitter. The glycine binding site on NMDA receptors is unaffected by strychnine and is, therefore, distinct from the glycine binding sites on previously described glycine receptors.

There may be an anatomical distinction between glycine inhibitory receptors and NMDA receptors. Glycine inhibitory receptors are most prominent in the spinal cord, with highest concentration in the corticospinal tract. NMDA receptors

Figure 9-3 The NMDA Receptor. *Allosteric stimulators are designated by + and allosteric inhibitors are designated by − . PCP is phencyclidine. Ca⁺⁺, Na⁺, and K⁺ can all move through the channel when it is open, but the entry of Ca⁺⁺ produces the greatest activation effect within the cell. (Modified from Olney, J.W. 1990. Excitotoxic amino acids and neuropsychiatric disorders. Ann. Rev. Pharmacol. 30:1–45.)*

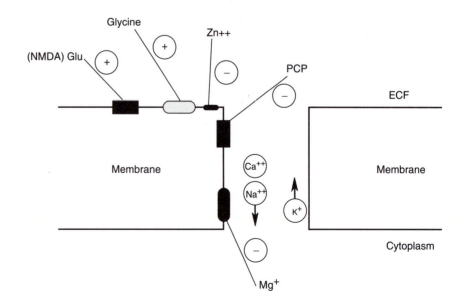

are predominantly found in the cerebral hemispheres, with an especially high density in certain areas involved in learning and memory, such as the hippocampus.

NMDA receptors allow cations such as Na^+ to pass through them. They, however, are commonly thought of as Ca^{++} channels. Since the Ca^{++} gradient across the membrane is quite high, in the range of 10^4, this calcium flux produces a strong depolarization (i.e., activation) of the cell. NMDA receptor depolarization is greater than that produced by the activation of other receptors, and is possibly the greatest that these cells normally experience.

NMDA receptors are well known for their ability to generate pathology and even to cause cell death. This is the phenomenon called "excitotoxicity." These unique receptors appear to be involved in the development of epileptic foci and may play a role in Alzheimer's disease as well as other pathological processes. Given this evidence, one is justified in asking, "What good are they?"

One possible major reason that evolution has selected for a high level of NMDA receptors is their possible role in learning, especially in the consolidation of long-term memory (Chapter 12). There has always been a fundamental question regarding the biochemistry of learning: "Given all the negative feedback controls in the brain, how does an organism override them at the molecular, cellular, and organ levels in order to learn?" Learning is fundamentally contrary to homeostasis and, as such, has been referred to by Jacques Barzun as being "against nature." In order for learning to take place, there must be some kind of mechanism, likely at the level of the cell, that overrides homeostasis and implants a new signal or code that can later be retrieved. NMDA receptors may provide that signal.

NMDA receptors have many properties that would be expected of a mechanism for establishing learning. They are able to depolarize cells to higher levels than normal, in fact requiring a "normal" depolarization before they are activated. They are therefore able to stimulate cells to high levels, and provide a mechanism whereby the cells can respond to more than one signal simultaneously. Thus, NMDA receptors are capable of overriding normal homeostatic forces, thereby establishing long-term memory. Unfortunately, such a mechanism also has the capability of producing pathology, even cell death. If activated inappropriately, NMDA receptors can cause the "learning" of undesirable characteristics (e.g., epilepsy). Thus, as with other important biological molecules, including oxygen and glucose, NMDA receptors are both necessary and potentially toxic. They must be carefully regulated, and drugs that interact with these receptors (either as agonists or antagonists) might be important tools for intervention. Such drugs are actively being sought.

SELF-STUDY QUESTIONS

Facts:

1. Which neurotransmitters use direct receptors?

2. What kind of ion channels produce ipsp's?

3. What kind of ion channels produce epsp's?

Concepts:

1. If direct receptors are analogous to allosteric enzymes, what reactions do the receptors catalyze?

2. Explain how an antagonist at a transmitter binding site can produce an excitatory effect on a cell.

BIBLIOGRAPHY

Biggio, G., and Costa, E., eds. 1990. GABA and benzodiazepine receptor subtypes. In *Advances in Biochemical Psychopharmacology*, edited by E. Costa and P. Greengard. New York: Raven Press.

Gasic, G.P., and Hollmann, M. 1992. Molecular neurobiology of glutamate receptors. *Ann. Rev. Physiol.* 54: 507–536.

Watkins, J.C., Krogsgaard-Larsen, P., and Honoré, T. 1990. Excitatory amino acid receptors. *Trends in Pharmacological Sciences*, 11: 25–33.

Sroblewski, J.T., and Danysz, W. 1989. Modulation of glutamate receptors: Molecular mechanisms and functional implications. *Ann. Rev. Pharmacol. Toxicol.* 29: 441–474.

CHAPTER 10

Fundamentals of Vision Biochemistry

OVERVIEW

In recent years, as more has been discovered about the molecular mechanisms of visual transduction, it has become clear that it is a model for many other kinds of signal transduction. Although the regulatory processes in vision are probably as complex as those in any system in the body, the molecular focus of this transduction system is very similar to that of many indirect receptors. Therefore, the general discussion of signal transduction begins with visual transduction.

Current estimates indicate that as much as a third of the total human brain cortex is involved with the processing of visual information, making vision arguably the most important of all the senses. The retina in the eye is the only part of the CNS directly visible from outside the body. The eye's function, transducing information in the form of light into physiologically and biochemically meaningful information, has long fascinated biological scientists. These factors make vision physiology and chemistry a highly specialized, prominent, and complex branch of neurochemistry.

Figure 10-1 shows a schema of the eye, illustrating that photons of light must traverse the entire eye before reaching the retina. The main functional cells in the retina are photoreceptor cells and many kinds of neurons, through which the retina communicates with the rest of the CNS. The principal photoreceptor cells are rods and cones. Rods are primarily responsive to low levels of ambient light or possibly to black and white information (purple absorption). The cones, which are further subdivided into three or more different kinds (red, green, and blue), are specialized for color vision.

Research on the cones in the retina, although increasing, lags behind that on rods. Rods are more numerous than cones and cover a larger surface area of the retina. Rods therefore constitute the bulk of the eye's light transducer cells. Rods are thus easier to isolate in sufficient quantity for scientific study. What holds true for rods appears, in general, also to be true for cones, with only small differences observed so far. This discussion, therefore, will focus on rods, with specific mention of cones when appropriate.

Rods are located at the "back" (dorsum) of the eye. This is the surface farthest from the site of light's entry, at the pupil. Rods are also at the "back" (most

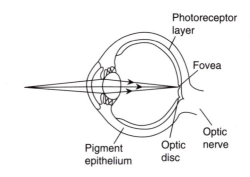

**Figure 10-1 The Eye
and Its Photoreceptors**

dorsal aspect) of the retina itself. Therefore, all impinging photons must traverse all other retinal cells before reaching the site of reception.

Figure 10-2 illustrates the anatomy of a rod, showing the rod's inner segment (RIS), the rod's outer segment (ROS), and the structure that connects them. The rod cell is like a neuron in many ways but is significantly different in others. It is a primary receptor cell, which neurons are not. It releases a transmitter that is inhibitory to postsynaptic cells. The transmitter, unexpectedly, is glutamate. This is the only context in which glutamate is known to be an inhibitory transmitter. Presumably, there is an as yet undescribed postsynaptic inhibitory receptor for glutamate.

Some anatomical peculiarities of rods are the location of mitochondria, the location of the Na^+K^+ATPases, and the presence of a large number of specialized discs. Both mitochondria and the Na^+K^+ATPases are specific to the RIS. There is a baseline depolarization of rod cells, in which Na^+ ions cross the plasma membrane into the cell in large quantities. This occurs predominantly in the ROS. Since the enzyme for extrusion of Na^+ back into the extracellular fluid is in the RIS, there is a continuous flow of Na^+ ions within the cell, from the outer to the inner segment. Flow, therefore, must also occur in the opposite direction in the extracellular fluid. The concentration of mitochondria in the inner segment is, at

**Figure 10-2 The
Structure of Rods
and Cones**

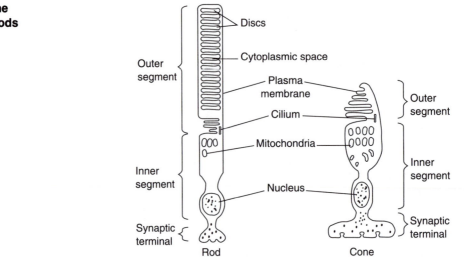

least in part, necessary to provide fuel for this massive pumping of ions back across the plasma membrane. Mitochondria are not known to be present in the ROS, which raises many questions about the energy supply to this aspect of the cell's activities.

The discs (Figure 10-2) in the outer segment move slowly but continuously outward from the RIS. The discs are apparently sloughed off from the cell, in the direction of the nearby pigment epithelium (PE) (Figure 10-1), with the macromolecules being digested by the lysosomal activity of PE cells.

While discs are within the rod cell they are the sites of transduction of light information into chemical signals. The discs take up the bulk of the volume of the outer segment and comprise over 95 percent of the total membranes of the ROS. They are formed from invaginations of the plasma membrane (an ongoing process, which occurs near the cilium). As the discs pinch off from the plasma membrane, they maintain the normal topology of endocytosis. That is, the sugar residues of glycosylated molecules remain in the lumen of the disc. The cytoplasmic surface of the discs, in common with the cytoplasmic surface of the plasma membrane, is not significantly glycosylated. The disc membrane itself is unusual in its fluidity: it has roughly the viscosity of olive oil. This fluidity is important for the function of the discs, and it is maintained, in part, by the large concentration of highly unsaturated fatty acids in the disc membrane. The retina has the highest concentration of docosahexaenoic acid (a fatty acid with sixteen carbons and six double bonds) in the body.

VISUAL TRANSDUCTION

Disc membranes are the actual site of visual transduction. The process begins with rhodopsin, a glycoprotein integral to the disc membrane. Rhodopsin has many properties in common with postsynaptic receptors, although it is receptive to a photon rather than a molecule. It is a member of a class of receptors sometimes called the "rhodopsin family." This family has become so large, with the recent discovery and cloning of many transmitter receptors, that it is now more frequently referred to as the **heptahelical** family of receptors. As this name implies, rhodopsin and the other members of the family have seven helices in their structure, each of which spans the membrane in which the receptor resides (Figure 10-3).

A significant portion of the structure of rhodopsin receptors is in the lumen of the disc. This includes the N-terminal portion, and it contains all the protein's glycosylation (CHO in Figure 10-3). The portion of the receptor in the cytoplasm is the C terminus. Many C-terminal residues have functional and/or regulatory roles in the mechanism of rhodopsin action. Besides the two terminals, both aqueous compartments also contain a few amino acids from the loops that connect the alpha helices (Figure 10-3). These loops, especially on the cytoplasmic side, also contain functional and regulatory groups.

The protein component of rhodopsin, as is the case in many receptors, is analogous in several ways to enzymes, and especially to allosteric enzymes. For example, some receptors require a hapten, or a cofactor, as many enzymes do. In the case of rhodopsin, the cofactor is a small lipid, 11 *cis* retinal. Retinal is an aldehyde derivative of vitamin A. It can be produced either from vitamin A or from

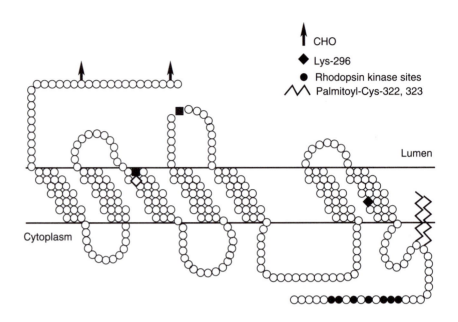

↑ CHO
◆ Lys-296
● Rhodopsin kinase sites
⋀⋀ Palmitoyl-Cys-322, 323

Lumen

Cytoplasm

**Figure 10-3 The
Structure of Rhodopsin**

beta carotene, the yellow pigment in vegetables such as carrots and sweet potatoes. The retinal cofactor is attached, by means of a Schiff base, to a lysine residue in the seventh helix of the rhodopsin, counting from the N-terminal. This location places the lipid group within the membrane (lys-296 in Figure 10-3). Either retinal or a closely related molecule is the chemical site of visual absorption in all visual species and in all visual cells. All three phyla on earth that have evolved visual receptors have independently settled on the same absorbing group. The specific wavelength absorbed by the visual pigment is determined by the combination of the absorption spectrum of the retinal and that of the protein to which it is attached. For example, rods and the three types of cones each absorb different wavelengths of photons, despite the fact that they all use the same retinal cofactor. Each cell has a different protein attached to the retinal. Although the four proteins are quite similar to each other, they vary somewhat in primary structure and therefore have different light absorptivities.

LIGHT RECEPTION

Response to Dark

The plasma membrane of the rod is depolarized by a continuous large flux of Na^+ and Ca^{++} ions into the cytoplasm. This flux is through a specialized channel, which is allosterically regulated by cytoplasmic cyclic GMP (cGMP).

The Na^+ ions entering the cell are later extruded by enzymes in the RIS, as discussed above. In this depolarized state, the rod releases large amounts of its inhibitory transmitter (i.e., glutamate) and tonically inhibits its postsynaptic cells.

Response to Light

The specific site of photon absorption is the double bond between carbons 11 and 12 of retinal. In rhodopsin this bond maximally absorbs photons of about 500 nm. Among other things, the photon's energy converts this bond from a *cis* to a *trans* double bond. There is also a slow separation of the all-*trans* retinal from the protein moiety, called opsin.

There are several different conformational states of rhodopsin that arise during the response to photon absorption. These have been characterized by quick freezing and other techniques. Of these successive forms, one called metarhodopsin II appears to be the biologically active molecule. While retaining both the retinal group and the energy of the photon, metarhodopsin II allosterically activates the next protein in the sequence. Figure 10-4 depicts a metarhodopsin II (designated R*) in the disc membrane. Associated with the membrane, on the cytoplasmic surface, are complexes of transducin (Ts) and phosphodiesterase (PDE). The edge of the disc membrane approaches the plasma membrane, which contains the Na^+Ca^{++} depolarizing channel. The cytoplasm between the two membranes contains soluble cyclic GMP, which is both the allosteric activator of the Na^+Ca^{++} channel and the substrate for the PDE.

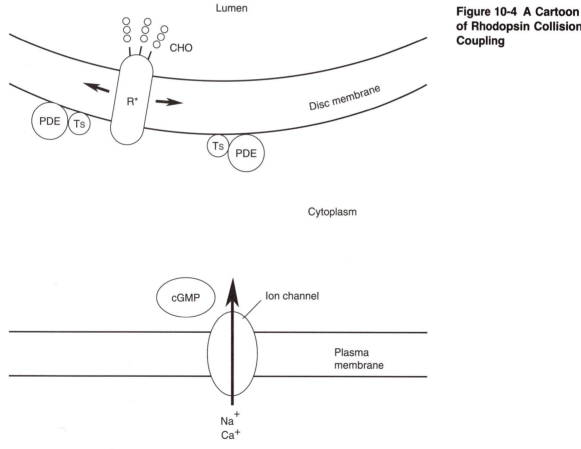

Figure 10-4 A Cartoon of Rhodopsin Collision Coupling

R*: Metarhodopsin II (activated rhodopsin)
Ts : Transducin, a G protein
cGMP : 3', 5' cyclic guanosine monophosphate
PDE : Phosphodiesterase
CHO : Carbohydrate portion of the rhodopsin glycoprotein

Because of the fluidity of the disc membrane, the several forms of rhodopsin (and most likely other proteins as well) move freely in the plane of the membrane. Rhodopsin traverses the membrane and has extensions on both sides, and this mobility allows it to interact with other proteins on either side of the membrane. This aspect of receptor interaction is sometimes called "collision coupling," because the activated receptor (e.g., metarhodopsin II) is able to collide with a number of other proteins associated with the membrane. If the receptor strikes another molecule that is able to respond allosterically, it is activated by the collision.

The next protein in rhodopsin's reaction sequence is a G protein. G proteins are a class of proteins with similar characteristics; the one in the rod cell is named transducin, because of its involvement in transducing light energy into chemical energy. The activated transducin, in turn, allosterically activates the PDE.

G proteins are highly speciaized allosteric enzymes that hydrolyze GTP. Different G proteins are involved in the regulation of a wide variety of cellular processes, including genomic expression and protein synthesis as well as receptor transduction. Some G proteins are inhibitory in function (and are called Gi), others are stimulatory (and are called **Gs**), and there are still others with different designations. All of these are specialized enzymes whose substrate is GTP. G proteins hydrolyze the GTP to GDP and inorganic phosphate. G proteins are unusual enzymes in that their catalyzed reaction is quite slow compared to other enzyme reactions, and the regulatory properties of the enzyme–substrate complex are thought of as being more important than the enzymatic reaction. The time required for transducin to hydrolyze its GTP substrate can be thought of as a timing mechanism for receptor action. As long as GTP is bound to the enzyme's active center, unhydrolyzed, the complex is able to activate allosterically the next protein in the sequence. As soon as the enzyme has hydrolyzed its substrate, and the active site contains GDP rather than GTP, the enzyme is no longer able to activate the next enzyme. This is the timing mechanism for the receptor's response.

In the case of rhodopsin, the transducin–GTP complex activates a phosphodiesterase (PDE) enzyme complex. The PDE is also associated with the disc membrane on the cytoplasmic side. This PDE is specific for cyclic GMP (cGMP), which is normally present in high concentration in the cytoplasm of the ROS. (The cGMP is the allosteric activator of the cation channel in the plasma membrane of the ROS.) The opening of this Na^+ and Ca^{++} channel maintains the rod in a depolarized state, in the dark.

This overall chain of events includes a series of allosteric activations, resulting in the closing of the cation (Na^+ and Ca^{++}) channels by the lowering of cGMP. Rhodopsin, in its activated, metarhodopsin II form, allosterically activates the Gs protein (transducin). Transducin, in turn, when it has a GTP bound to it, activates the PDE. The activated PDE reduces the concentration of cGMP, which is the allosteric activator of the channel, thereby decreasing cation permeability at the plasma membrane.

The result of all this is that a single photon, activating a single molecule of rhodopsin to metarhodopsin II, is capable in theory of activating all the transducin molecules on a single disc by collision coupling. This, in turn, could activate all the PDEs associated with that disc. As the PDEs reduce the cGMP concentration in the cytosol, the cation channels in the plasma membrane admit fewer cations, and the cell's depolarization is lessened.

This biochemical process decreases the activation of the cell, and is therefore in the direction of a hyperpolarization. The hyperpolarization decreases the amount of transmitter released by the rod and therefore decreases the extent to which the postsynaptic cells are inhibited. Because it decreases inhibition, this response is an activation. In fact, a dark-adapted rod cell can produce a measurable change in rod activity in response to a single photon.

THE RESTORATION OF RHODOPSIN

A question can be raised by the above sequence of events: "How is the rhodopsin molecule recycled, since it was covalently modified during its response to light?" At the end of its response, as described above, the retinal cofactor was in the all-*trans* form and was separate from the opsin protein moiety.

Over the years, several different hypotheses regarding the mechanism of the recycling process (some involving organs as far away as the liver) have been proposed. Currently, most attention is given to two hypotheses, in one of which the pigment epithelium (PE) participates. In this proposal, either the retinal cofactor is restored to its 11-*cis* form or a new vitamin A molecule is converted into active retinal in the pigment epithelium. In either case, the retinal cofactor is attached to an opsin in the PE, from which it is recycled to the nearby ROS.

Another hypothesis involves two enzymes discovered within the rod cell itself. This system requires the participation of the phospholipid, phosphatidyl ethanolamine (PE). All-*trans* retinal is enzymatically attached to a molecule of PE as a Schiff base. This retinal complex absorbs photons at a different wavelength from those absorbed by rhodopsin or the other protein pigments in the retina. When the PE–*trans* retinal complex absorbs a photon, the retinal cofactor is converted back to the 11-*cis* form in a non-enzymatic reaction. The restored retinal is then enzymatically transferred from the lipid back to opsin, recreating active rhodopsin, in situ. This pathway has the virtue of being entirely within the ROS.

OTHER MECHANISMS FOR REGULATION OF RHODOPSIN

In addition to the regulatory activities discussed above, other systems of regulation of rhodopsin exist, at different levels of organization. In the predominantly allosteric system discussed above, the activity of rhodopsin is slowly reduced by the loss of its retinal group (now changed in structure) and by the hydrolysis of GTP molecules on transducin. Another important means by which down regulation of rhodopsin activity occurs is phosphorylation, in this case catalyzed by a kinase physically associated with it.

The activity of allosteric proteins is often modified by the enzymatic addition of phosphate groups to specific regulatory sites within the protein. Receptors of the rhodopsin, or heptahelical, family are usually regulated in this way as well. Most commonly, regulatory phosphorylation occurs on cytoplasmic portions of the molecule, on serine or threonine residues. The most common sites for such regulation are serines and threonines in the cytoplasmic C-terminal sequence and the last, or third, amino acid loop, the one connecting the sixth and seventh helices (Figure 10-3). Phosphorylation at these sites often inhibits the receptor from responding to its activator. These phosphorylations are catalyzed by one or more specific protein kinases, which may be directly associated with the rhodopsin molecule. In fact, many transmitter receptors may have such associated protein kinases, physically ready to phosphorylate the receptor and down regulate its activity. Since this kind of regulation is a covalent modification, it is more long-lasting than the allosteric effects mentioned above. Later, a phosphatase is necessary to remove the phosphate group and restore the receptor to the resting state.

SELF-STUDY QUESTIONS

Facts:

1. What are the anatomical and cellular locations of the functional aspects of the visual system?

2. What is the specific function of each component of the rod's light responsiveness in light transduction?

3. How is rhodopsin restored after being used for signal transduction?

Concepts:

1. Describe the concept of collision coupling.

2. Describe the role of cGMP in light transduction.

BIBLIOGRAPHY

Hubbell, W.L., and Bownds, M.D. 1979. Visual transduction in vertebrate photoreceptors. *Annual Review of Neuroscience* 2:17–34.

Nathans, J. 1987. Molecular biology of visual pigments. *Annual Review of Neuroscience* 10:163–194.

Shichi, H. 1989. Molecular biology of vision. In *Basic Neurochemistry*, edited by G. Siegel, B. Agranoff, R.W. Albers, and P. Molinoff. New York: Raven Press.

CHAPTER 11

Indirect Receptors and Second Messenger Systems

The term indirect receptor is used here to refer to those receptors that are linked to a "second messenger" system. Many are also linked to G proteins, discussed below. Some of these are sometimes called "metabotropic" receptors. These receptors respond to a ligand, such as a neurotransmitter, by increasing the formation of one or more small, diffusible molecules, called second messengers. These messengers are allosteric effectors (i.e., either activators or inhibitors) of other regulatory processes. Although the diffusible molecule may not be the second in the sequence, the term "second messenger" has become permanently attached to this group of regulators.

The best-characterized second messengers are $3',5'$ cyclic adenosine monophosphate (cAMP), $3',5'$ cyclic guanosine monophosphate (cGMP), inositol 1,4,5 trisphosphate (IP3), diacylglycerol (DAG), eicosanoids (e.g., prostaglandins and other molecules made from arachidonic acid), Ca^{++}, and Ca^{++} complexed to **calmodulin** (Ca-CM). Nitric oxide, a small, diffusible molecule of considerable biological importance, might also be considered a second messenger. All of these are powerful regulatory molecules or complexes capable of modifying the activity of one or more enzymes, cytoskeletal elements, genomic proteins, ion channels, and other functional proteins. The concentration of each is increased in response to one or more receptors, and they can therefore be considered second messengers. Other substances are sometimes called second messengers, including such complex structures as the G proteins themselves, but the term is most commonly applied to these relatively small, diffusible molecules.

OVERVIEW

Receptors that use second messengers require a longer time than direct receptors to produce their effects (milliseconds to seconds, as opposed to microseconds), because of the time required for the requisite sequence of reactions. In some cases, the sequence is quite lengthy, involving different cellular compartments. Unlike direct receptors, however, second messenger systems are often associated with a signal amplification mechanism that allows each molecule of transmitter to have greatly magnified effects.

The earliest-known indirect receptor is rhodopsin (Chapter 10). It is the prototype for the heptahelical (i.e., seven transmembrane helices) family of receptors, the largest known class of indirect receptors. All members of this family have seven transmembrane alpha helices and have their N terminals in the extracellular space and their C terminals in the cytoplasm. All have glycosylation restricted to the N-terminal portion of the molecule and are reversibly phosphorylated on the C-terminal section in the cytoplasm. Many also have reversible phosphorylation sites on the third intracellular loop (Figure 11-1). These phosphorylation sites, for regulation of the receptor's activity, are important to the overall function. Phosphorylations may occur at other locations, but the intracellular portions of the molecule appear to contain the majority of such sites. The C-terminal region, in many cases, also contains one or more sites where hydrophobic groups may be attached. These attachments are often at the -SH group of the amino acid cysteine, and include such residues as fatty acids or **isoprenyl** groups. The hydrophobic groups may serve to bind the C-terminal portion of the receptor protein molecule to the cytoplasmic surface of the membrane, as well as having other functions.

The third cytoplasmic loop (in the cytoplasm of the recipient cell) is also the site of interaction between the receptor and the next protein in the response sequence, the G protein enzyme (Figures 11-2, opposite, and 10-4, page 103). G proteins are roughly subdivided into several subclasses. Two important subclasses are Gi and Gs. Gi proteins inhibit the next molecule in the sequence, and Gs proteins stimulate the next enzyme (see Figures 10-4, 11-2, and 11-4). Finally, some of these heptahelical, transmembrane receptor molecules have some of the properties of a channel. For example, after being activated by absorbing a photon, rhodopsin allows protons to move across the membrane.

Figure 11-1 Beta-2
Adrenergic Receptor

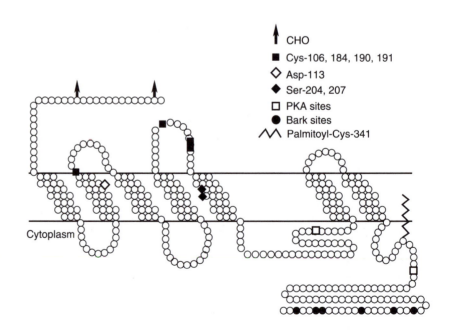

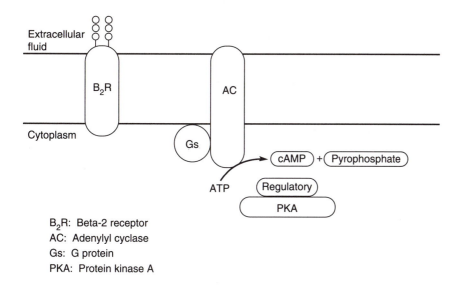

B₂R: Beta-2 receptor
AC: Adenylyl cyclase
Gs: G protein
PKA: Protein kinase A

Figure 11-2 The Cellular Machinery for a Beta Receptor's Response to Binding NE

HEPTAHELICAL RECEPTORS

Besides rhodopsin, other receptors belonging to the heptahelical receptor family are the muscarinic acetylcholine receptors (several of which have now been cloned and sequenced); noradrenaline (norepinephrine) receptors (both the alpha and beta subclasses have been expanded to several members each); dopamine and serotonin receptors (of which there are at least five each); and the receptors for at least two peptide transmitters, substance P and substance K. The metabotropic excitatory amino acid receptors and the GABA-B receptor also likely belong to this family.

The heptahelical family of receptors, in common with direct receptors, responds to the binding of the appropriate ligand with an (allosteric) conformational change. That is, the receptor with the transmitter bound to it has a different three-dimensional shape from the unbound form. This change of conformation is the basis for the allosteric interaction with the next molecule in line, and so on through the entire sequence.

One of the most intensively studied members of the heptahelical family of neurotransmitter receptors is the noradrenaline (NE) beta-2 receptor (Figure 11-1). It has been cloned, sequenced, and reconstituted in vitro. Its particular biochemical properties have been studied by synthesizing mutations containing modified or substitute amino acids. It now serves as the model for the other members of the family. The NE beta-2 receptor binds NE within the membrane, at a site that is close to the extracellular surface but not wholly exposed to it. There is some evidence that this binding requires the aid of a lipid molecule with **amphoteric** properties.

Although it is controversial, there is also evidence that the occupied receptor activates nearby enzymes that are closely associated with the membrane, and that these enzymes convert phospholipids into forms that increase membrane mobility.

In any case, once the receptor is occupied, it has the ability to move laterally in the plane of the membrane. This ability is analogous to the situation with activated rhodopsin.

The moving complex of receptor and ligand is now free to participate in collision coupling by interacting with protein complexes on the cytoplasmic surface of the membrane. This is possible because the receptor traverses the membrane, having extensions on both surfaces. When G proteins are encountered on the cytoplasmic surface, the G protein can be allosterically modified by the collision. As mentioned, the binding between the G protein and the receptor appears to be primarily at the third intracellular loop of the receptor. This interaction, in fact, can be prevented by phosphorylation of specific sites on the third loop. The resulting phosphate groups may be near the G protein binding site, and therefore could directly interfere with the binding. Some psychotropic drugs (for example, lithium) may work in a similar way, by binding to either one or the other protein and interfering with the receptor–G protein interaction. In any case, binding between the NE beta-2 receptor complex and its receptive G protein is specific, and is therefore a site for drug intervention.

The G protein is an enzyme (with a very slow velocity), and when it is activated by binding to the receptor complex, its Km for GTP is lowered, while that for GDP is raised. Thus, as the G protein binds a GTP, the resulting G protein–GTP complex becomes an allosteric effector. This complex, in a cell containing beta-2 receptors, activates an adenylyl cyclase, also associated with the membrane. Adenylyl cyclase, when activated, binds ATP in the cytoplasm of the cell, as a substrate, and produces cAMP. The cAMP is itself, in turn, an allosteric activator of cyclic AMP–dependent protein kinase (also called protein kinase A, or PKA). PKA is not associated with the membrane, but is free in the cytoplasm. It is therefore able to phosphorylate a large number of different substrates in diverse cellular compartments. PKA substrates include metabolic enzymes, cytoskeletal elements, membrane molecules such as ion channels, and regulatory proteins in the cell's genome.

The entire system, by which the neurotransmitter effects postsynaptic changes, thus includes a minimum of five different functional proteins, in addition to the small molecules (NE, GTP, and ATP):

1. The receptor: The protein molecule that binds the transmitter, undergoes conformational changes, and becomes an allosteric effector while the transmitter is bound to it
2. The G protein: Actually a multiple polypeptide complex (alpha, beta, and gamma), which is allosterically activated to bind and hydrolyze GTP. (As is true of all triphosphatases, it is a Mg^{++} requiring enzyme.) The slow rate of this hydrolysis (i.e., the time during which a GTP is bound to the G protein) is the time during which the complex of G alpha and GTP is allosterically active.
3. Adenylyl cyclase: The enzyme activated by the G alpha–GTP complex
4. Protein kinase A: The enzyme activated by the product of the adenylyl cyclase reaction (i.e., cAMP)
5. One or more various proteins phosphorylated by protein kinase A

The length of this sequence partially explains the time required for indirect receptors to act. If one of the final protein substrates of PKA is an ion channel, at least four allosteric steps must occur in sequence before the channel's permeability is changed. Direct receptors can effect ion permeability changes within microseconds, whereas second messenger systems sometimes require seconds before their full effects are achieved.

The overall amplification factor in this sequence can be enormous. One NE molecule, bound to one receptor, can activate as many G proteins as it is able to encounter. Each G protein can activate at least one adenylyl cyclase for a period of time. During that time, each adenylyl cyclase can produce hundreds to thousands of cAMP molecules. The cAMP can activate a PKA, on a more or less one-to-one basis, and each PKA can phosphorylate tens to hundreds of proteins. Therefore, a single NE molecule, at least in theory, is able to generate multiple thousands of phosphorylations in diverse locations in the cell, within milliseconds to seconds of its being presynaptically released.

Desensitization

Second messenger receptor systems also undergo desensitization, a similar mechanism to that observed with direct receptors. Phosphorylation of the receptor molecule can produce a temporary inhibition, lasting as long as the phosphate group remains attached. As mentioned, phosphorylation sites are cytoplasmic, mostly in the C-terminal sequence. Beta-2 adrenergic receptors, for example, are substrates for a specific kinase, beta adrenergic receptor kinase (or BARK). The occupation of the receptor by NE allosterically activates BARK, which then phosphorylates the receptor. The phosphorylated receptor complex is sequestered within the cell, and thereby inactivated for a longer period of time. Therefore, the receptor–NE complex is able to activate G proteins only during the time prior to its phosphorylation and sequestration. Each receptor molecule, of all types studied so far, has multiple phosphorylation sites. Different protein kinases have different specificities for some sites. An individual protein, subject to regulation by phosphorylation, may have more than a dozen different phosphorylation sites, each of which may produce somewhat different effects.

Another well-studied receptor in this class, rhodopsin, is also subject to desensitization by phosphorylation. This step is catalyzed by a specific rhodopsin kinase, which similarly inactivates the molecule. In both these cases, the kinase is tightly associated with the receptor. In fact, some early attempts to purify the receptor resulted in retention of the kinase.

OTHER SECOND MESSENGERS OF THE HEPTAHELICAL RECEPTOR FAMILY

Although all known members of the heptahelical receptor family couple to G proteins, their G proteins are not all alike: they do not all affect the same enzymes and they do not all use the same second messengers. Rhodopsin's G protein activates a phosphodiesterase and reduces the concentration of cGMP. The NE beta-2 receptor activates adenylyl cyclase and increases the concentration of cAMP. Many of the acetylcholine muscarinic receptors and serotonin receptors (e.g., 5-HT1c and 5-HT2) affect a G protein that activates a phospholipase C (PLC).

There are many phospholipases in living systems. These are enzymes that hydrolyze one of the bonds in a phospholipid. When these hydrolases were first discovered, they were given different letters to designate the bond in the phospholipid for which they were specific. Figure 11-3 shows the structure of a particular phospholipid. Phospholipases A hydrolyze fatty acids from the glycerol moiety, A1 from the number 1 position and A2 from the second position. Phospholipase C is the designation for enzymes that hydrolyze the bond between the phosphate group and the third carbon of the glycerol. Breaking any phospholipid at this point produces a diacylglycerol (DAG) and a small, water-soluble alcohol with the phosphate group still attached. Phospholipase D is used for enzymes that hydrolyze the bond between the phosphate and the remaining hydrophilic moiety.

The DAG moiety has physical properties similar to cholesterol. It is hydrophobic. It contains two fatty acid chains in ester linkage. Therefore, once it is formed, it remains associated with the hydrophobic membrane. The only hydrophilic portion of a DAG is the free hydroxyl group, previously esterified to phosphate.

The nature of the small, hydrophilic phosphate residue that is separated from the DAG depends on the specific phospholipid attacked by the phospholipase. In producing second messengers, the best-known substrate for PLC is phosphoinositol bisphosphate, PIP2 (Figure 11-3). In this case, the hydrophilic residue released is IP3, or inositol 1,4,5 trisphosphate. A molecule of this size with three charged phosphate groups is intensely hydrophilic. IP3 moves into the cytoplasm after its release from PIP2 in the membrane. Thus, in a single enzymatic reaction, two different second messengers have been produced in two different cellular compartments (the cytoplasmic surface of the plasma membrane and within the cytoplasm). Figure 11-4 illustrates the reaction.

DAG allosterically activates a protein kinase C (PKC). The PKC is also associated with the cytoplasmic surface of the plasma membrane. PKCs are a

Figure 11-3 The structure of phosphoinositol bisphosphate, showing points where phospholipases hydrolyze a phospholipid. (Letters stand for phospholipid designation).

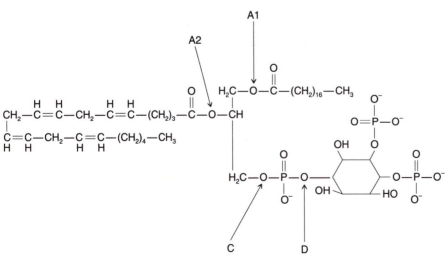

Extracellular fluid

113

*Other Second
Messengers of the
Heptahelical Receptor
Family*

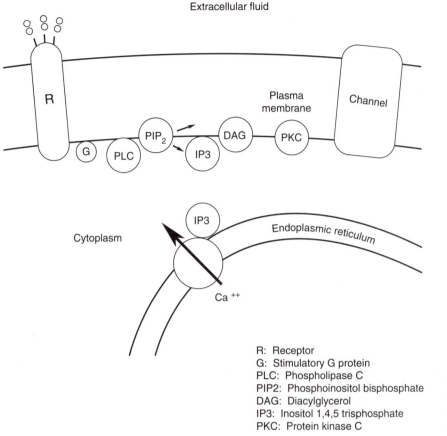

R: Receptor
G: Stimulatory G protein
PLC: Phospholipase C
PIP2: Phosphoinositol bisphosphate
DAG: Diacylglycerol
IP3: Inositol 1,4,5 trisphosphate
PKC: Protein kinase C

**Figure 11-4 The
Phosphoinositide
Second Messenger
System**

family of enzymes, designated C for historical reasons. There are several different specific PKCs, but activation by a DAG and association with membranes are properties that many of them share.

Because of its membrane location, the PKC is expected to act upon substrates that are also in or near the membrane. In fact, many PKC substrates may be ion channels, where their cytoplasmic portions could be phosphorylated by PKC. As the channels are themselves allosteric proteins, such a phosphorylation can be expected to modify the channels' ion permeability properties. PKCs, like PKAs, may also phosphorylate the receptor molecules that began the process of activating them, thereby establishing a negative feedback loop.

The IP3 that is released into the cytoplasm by PLC is also an allosteric effector. It binds to a Ca^{++} channel and allosterically causes it to open. In this case, the affected Ca^{++} channel is in the membrane of the endoplasmic reticulum (ER), inside the cell. IP3 diffuses through the cytoplasm and is therefore able to migrate a significant distance from the site of its production. Upon activating the Ca^{++} channels in the ER, Ca^{++} enters the cytoplasm from the lumen of the ER (where its concentration may be as high as that in extracellular fluid). Extracellular Ca^{++} is normally in the millimolar range, whereas cytoplasmic Ca^{++} is usually submicromolar. The Ca^{++} concentration gradient into the cytoplasm is of the order of 10^4 or greater. Since the total pool of Ca^{++} is large in the ER, a significant change in cytoplasmic Ca^{++} concentration can occur in response to a small number of IP3s.

There has been considerable interest in studying the metabolism of IP3 and related inositol phosphates. There are relatively specific enzymes that both phosphorylate and dephosphorylate these inositol derivates, changing the biological activity markedly with each change of phosphorylation. Changes in the activities of these enzymes can therefore affect the function of transmitters that use IP3 as a second messenger. There is speculation that lithium's effectiveness as a psychotropic drug occurs in this system. Lithium is an inhibitor of many phosphatases, and its presence will therefore increase the concentrations of some inositol phosphates.

Ca^{++} can also be thought of as a second messenger. Ca^{++}, alone or in combination with calmodulin, can affect a large number of cellular processes, most of which are excitatory. Therefore, transmitters that use the IP3/DAG second messenger system are excitatory, at least with respect to Ca^{++} concentration in the postsynaptic cell.

High calcium concentration in the cytoplasm of cells is capable of more than just excitation, however. Too high a concentration of calcium in cells is a part of the cytotoxicity mechanism, and can be lethal. The extent to which IP3 from heptahelical receptor activity might be lethal is not presently known.

OTHER TYPES OF INDIRECT RECEPTORS

In addition to the heptahelical family of receptors, which use G proteins and affect virtually all cell processes, there are other types of indirect receptors. The best-characterized class of these is the membrane-bound guanylyl cyclases. These enzymes are integral membrane proteins that span the membrane in which they reside. Figure 11-5 is a diagram of a guanylyl cyclase. The "receptor" and the "effector" part of the receptor system may be thought of as being combined. The

Figure 11-5 A Cartoon of a Membrane Guanylyl Cyclase

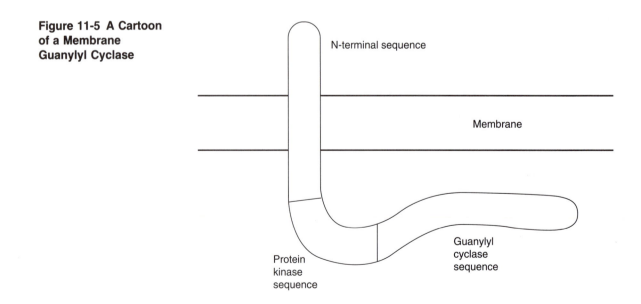

portion of the protein in the extracellular fluid (i.e., the glycosylated part) binds a transmitter or signal molecule (usually a peptide). The receptor is allosterically activated by the binding, causing the cytoplasmic portion to produce cGMP. In some membrane-bound guanylyl cyclases, the cytoplasmic portion of the molecule also contains a sequence that might either have protein kinase activity or be an inhibitor of protein kinases. In this case, the activation of the protein kinase may not require the presence of the cGMP. In any case, the biological roles of cGMP are less well understood than those of cAMP.

SELF-STUDY QUESTIONS

Facts:

1. Which transmitters use which second messengers?

2. In which compartment(s) does each second messenger operate?

3. Which enzymes or other proteins are affected by each second messenger system?

4. What do Gi and Gs stand for?

5. Outline the sequence of events that occurs after the binding of NE to a beta-2 receptor.

Concepts:

1. Discuss the interaction sites of heptahelical receptors with their G proteins.

2. What is the mechanism of action of Li^+?

3. Explain the amplification that occurs with transmitters that use heptahelical receptors.

BIBLIOGRAPHY

Berridge, M.J. 1987. Inositol trisphosphate and diacylglycerol: Two interacting second messengers. *Annual Review of Biochemistry* 56: 159–194.

Bourne, H., Sanders, D.A., and McCormick, F. 1991. The GTPase superfamily: Conserved structure and molecular mechanism. *Nature* 349: 117–127.

Chinkers, M., and Garbers, D.L. 1991. Signal transduction by guanylyl cyclases. *Annual Review of Biochemistry* 60: 553–575.

Dohlman, H.G., Thorner, J., Caron, M.G., and Lefkowitz, R.J. 1991. Model systems for the study of seven-transmembrane-segment receptors. *Annual Review of Biochemistry* 60: 653–688.

Majerus, P.W. 1992. Inositol phosphate biochemistry. *Annual Review of Biochemistry* 61: 225–250.

Organ Neurochemistry

CHAPTER 12

Learning and Memory

It is difficult to study learning without including memory, since memory is the product of the learning process. Therefore, it is common to consider them together. Learning has traditionally been defined by psychologists as "a modification of behavior as a result of experience." The definition's focus on behavior indicates the past dependence of most learning studies on observation of lower animals. Human studies, in which the subjects can communicate by a variety of means, have also provided considerable insight in recent years. The fundamental distinction—that learning is the process and memory is the product—persists, however, despite the increasing complexity of both areas of research.

Memory is the trace laid down in the brain that corresponds to a particular bit of learned information, and there have been many hypotheses about the nature of this trace. Whatever its nature, it is called an **engram.** One major hypothesis about the engram was formulated by D. O. Hebb, of McGill University. Hebb speculated that the engram was a synaptic network, possibly linking synapses and neurons throughout the brain for a particular learned bit of information. Current computer modeling and neural network theory about memory are based on this hypothesis, as is a majority of modern biological research on memory.

An alternative theory about the nature of memory, popular in the 1960s, was that an engram might be a molecule of some sort, usually thought of as either protein or RNA. This hypothesis generated quite a few highly publicized experiments, but their reproducibility was limited. The hypothesis does not currently have many supporters.

If the engram is indeed a synaptic network, a fundamental question remains about whether new synapses are made when something new is learned, or whether older synapses are remodeled to incorporate the new bit of knowledge, or both. In any case, the hypothesis requires that certain kinds of biochemical and physiological changes occur in and around synapses during learning. Some of these changes, or other changes initiated by them, must be at least semipermanent. Experiments based on this hypothesis have been fruitful and have produced results that fit well with chemical and physiological data from other sources.

The total amount of published information about learning and its mechanisms is quite large. Only a few selected experiments and observations are discussed here.

STAGES OF MEMORY

It has been convenient to separate the learning process into two stages, one producing short-term memory (STM) and one producing long-term memory (LTM). This is an oversimplification, as other logical stages are known to exist, but the distinction remains useful. An organism can learn a specific task, but if electrical shock or physical trauma (e.g., a blow to the head) intervenes within a certain period of time, the memory of the learning is forever lost. The major inference about the engram that arises from these observations is that knowledge can be stored as an electrical, not a chemical, activation of a synaptic network. That is, a temporary electrical activation of synapses is involved, but the structure of synapses is not changed. If one waits several minutes after learning, depending on the task or the species, the same shock or trauma will no longer eliminate what was learned. It is believed that with time the engram is encoded into molecular changes in the synaptic network, and that these changes have much greater staying power than the form that could be disrupted.

The easily disrupted form of knowledge is referred to as STM, and the more resistant form is called LTM. LTM is resistant to prolonged periods of **coma,** as well as to (brief) electrical "storms," such as epileptic seizures. The designations STM and LTM may be on the verge of being dropped because of increasing knowledge of the complexity of learning, but they will remain in use for some time outside the laboratories of researchers in this area. For LTM to form, an STM must be present in the brain. Therefore, LTM formation is sometimes referred to as "consolidation" of an STM into an LTM.

Researchers also divide learning into "non-associative" and "associative" forms. **Non-associative,** the simplest kind of learning, is further subdivided into "habituation" and "sensitization" (or potentiation). **Habituation** is the term given to the decrease in neuronal activity in response to repetitions of the same stimulus over time. This phenomenon can be studied in quite simple neural systems, even in single synapses involving only two cells. It has been shown to be produced by a diminution of the amount of transmitter released in response to a repeated stimulus. Less transmitter produces less of an effect on the postsynaptic cell(s), reducing the effect resulting from the stimulus. If the stimulus is continually repeated over the long term, a further decrease in response occurs, now due to changes in the synaptic structure. Specifically, some synapses are eliminated, leaving fewer possible sites for the postsynaptic effect. Although the inference that can be made from this observation is that the molecular mechanism of habituation is presynaptic, the details are not yet fully known. Habituation is homeostatic in direction, analogous to negative feedback inhibition of a metabolic pathway. It is a kind of learning and is possibly related to some higher learning processes. The ease of habituation of newborn humans has been shown to correlate to their subsequent IQ.

Sensitization is the opposite of habituation, in that there is an increase in neuronal activity in response to repeated stimulation over time. In this process, simple associations can be made and may even be required. Sensitization is not true associative learning because the **conditioned stimulus** does not eventually replace the **unconditioned stimulus.** In sensitization, the effects are algebraically additive. For example, consider the case of *Aplysia* (a mollusk also known as the California sea hare), studied by Eric Kandel and James Schwartz. The snail is initially stimulated in a relatively mild way (e.g., by squirting it with a stream of water). This causes the animal to retract its siphon, which is normally extended into the water as a food-gathering device. Repeated squirts of water result in a diminished siphon retraction, illustrating habituation. If, in addition to the water stream, the animal receives a noxious stimulus (e.g., a shock to the head), the response to the stream of water will be increased with time. The noxious stimulus need be given only once. Sensitization can reverse habituation completely, even if the animal has fully habituated prior to experiencing the noxious stimulus. As in habituation, the initial effect is produced by changes in the amount of neurotransmitter released in response to the stimulus. Again, if the animal is sensitized and stimulated chronically, the long-term effect is to change synaptic structure. In this case, new synapses are created, allowing a much greater postsynaptic response to a single presynaptic stimulus. (Figure 12-1 illustrates these structural changes.)

ASSOCIATIVE LEARNING

In recent years, primarily because of the work of Mortimer Mishkin and his colleagues, **associative** learning has been subdivided into **reflexive** learning (or habit) and **declarative** (or cognitive or higher) learning. Different terms are used for these classes, but the distinction is important. These two systems, apparently characteristic of primates and possibly of other higher mammals, are to some degree physically separated within the brain. The most important distinction, as implied by the designations, is that one system predominates in the learning that forms higher consciousness, and the other (habit) can take place free of cognition.

Mishkin's results indicate that reflexive learning more heavily involves nuclei in the brain stem, and that its acquisition is based primarily on repetition. Higher learning has been known for some time to require psychological "arousal"; it is not entirely clear whether reflexive learning does also. The dopaminergic system in the nigrostriatal tract may be requisite for reflexive learning and, if so, could be the arousal mechanism. Much of the psychological research on learning in the earlier part of this century, using the fundamental "stimulus-response" paradigm, was studying the reflexive system.

Figure 12-1 *Long-term habituation and sensitization are accompanied by structural changes in the presynaptic terminals of sensory neurons. Long-term habituation leads to a loss of synapses, long-term sensitization to an increase.*

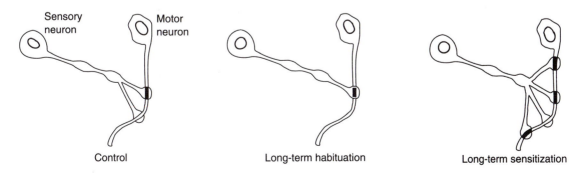

In addition to reflexive and declarative learning, higher kinds of cognitive learning can occur, including "meta" learning. Meta learning is learning "what one knows"—for example, "I know that I know my address and telephone number." Brain pathways for higher learning are much more complex than those for reflexive learning and involve portions of the limbic system, such as hippocampus, amygdala, dorsomedial thalamus, and ventromedial prefrontal cortex. As mentioned, higher learning does require some kind of arousal, and activation of the locus ceruleus (Chapter 6) is thought to be the arousal mechanism for this system.

In summary, an oversimplified categorization of learning breaks it down into non-associative and associative components. Non-associative learning is further broken down into habituation and sensitization. Associative learning is subdivided into reflexive and declarative learning. All of these can be subdivided into STM and LTM, depending solely on the length of time that separates the learned event from the formation of the engram.

ANATOMICAL REQUIREMENTS FOR HIGHER LEARNING

The special importance of the hippocampus in higher learning has been known for at least three decades. There have been a number of neurosurgical cases that make this point, including a famous one called "H.M.," but one particular patient can be considered a paradigm case. P.B. was a patient of Wilder Penfield in Montreal in the 1950s. He had serious, frequent seizures, and was treated with two separate neurosurgical procedures. During the second operation, the **anterior** half of one hippocampus was removed. The difference in the patient's functioning that resulted is well worth reviewing today. In 1973, Dr. Penfield came out of retirement to publish the autopsy findings. P.B. had no hippocampus in the **contralateral** hemisphere. Therefore, although the surgeons at the time were unaware of it, the second operation left P.B. with a bilateral anterior hippocampectomy (i.e., no anterior hippocampus on either side).

P.B. had an above-average IQ (about 120). He was a civil engineer and had been office manager in an engineering firm. He was unable to retain this position after his surgery. Although his IQ and his STM were intact, he was no longer able to form higher cognitive LTM. He was retained by the firm as a draftsman. Each morning he had to relearn the drawing he was working on. He could not take a significant break (i.e., interrupt his concentration on the project) without having to start over again. On the other hand, he was able to keep an individual project in mind for an entire working day if he did not break his concentration. He also, as a result of his inability to form new memory, had significant problems in his personal life, ranging from a damaged relationship with his fiancee to difficulty finding his way home after moving to a new house.

This latter point also illustrates the difference in the two learning systems in the brain. P.B. was able to learn how to get to his new home after many repetitions of the journey with help, but he did not learn that he knew it. If given a map of the city, he could not point out his dwelling. Thus, he was able to use the reflexive, or motor, pathway for learning the journey, but could not incorporate the meta knowledge that he knew it.

From the study of patient P.B. in combination with several other, similar patients, it is possible to conclude that the anterior half of at least one hippocampus is necessary for the consolidation of cognitive LTM. The case also demonstrates that there is a learning pathway for habit or repetitive actions that does not require the anterior hippocampus.

Clinical evidence has also implicated the dorsomedial nuclei of the thalamus (DMT) as being necessary for the formation of declarative LTM. This formation is damaged, bilaterally, in various disease states caused by a brain deficiency of thiamine. This deficiency is now called the Wernicke-Korsakoff syndrome. (Wernicke's encephalopathy and Korsakoff's psychosis are known to be associated.) The most common cause of this syndrome in the United States is alcoholism, although **hyperemesis** can also produce the disease. (Wernicke's first patient, in fact, was a young woman who suffered from excessive vomiting caused by her work conditions.) Irreversible, bilateral damage to the DMT also results in difficulty with new learning. Many of these patients, however, will show this symptom early enough in the course of their disease for the symptom to reverse if the causative factor is taken away (e.g., if the patient stops drinking). Discussion of bilateral damage to the mammillary bodies as a cause of Wernicke-Korsakoff syndrome has been widely published, but in a very large study of patients from Boston and Cleveland, the only neuropathology that correlated exactly with the impairment of new learning was bilateral degeneration of DMT. In all the above patients, STM formation was intact; the difficulty they experienced was a block in the consolidation of STM into LTM.

A final note about anatomy and learning ability relates to brain size. In the nineteenth and earlier twentieth centuries, there was a highly publicized debate about the relationship of IQ and head size. This debate, among other things, allowed some to argue that women were inferior to men, as the brains of women on average are 10 to 15 percent smaller than those of men. There is now considerable evidence that strongly refutes this contention. However, one anatomical finding that seems to correlate directly with IQ is total synaptic number. This number does not necessarily correlate with brain size, but it does seem to correlate with the size of certain portions of brain, for example, the cerebral cortex. The thickness of the cortical layer, at least in rodents in which it has been measured experimentally, correlates with the total number of synapses, as well as with the ability to perform well in mazes.

Further, the same experimenters who first studied this phenomenon in rodents also found that large differences in the level of stimulation in the early post-natal environment could produce large differences in synaptic number and cortical thickness. Rats raised in highly stimulating environments, with many objects and other rats to play with, developed thicker cortices and greater ability to negotiate mazes than litter mates raised in conditions affording little or no stimulation. It seems fair to conclude that, though gross brain size does not necessarily correlate with intelligence, total synaptic number does.

BIOCHEMICAL STUDIES OF LEARNING AND MEMORY

Anatomical correlates of intelligence underscore the importance of a biological, hence a biochemical, role in learning. Additional, much stronger data come from the study of genetics and IQ. A genetically controlled process is, by definition, a biochemical process, since genes are expressed chemically. There has been considerable controversy about the genetics of IQ, although much of the controversy is occurring outside of the scientific community. Many people on both sides of the debate appear to have a political agenda, but two clear scientific conclusions emerge from the data.

It is true that there is a strong genetic component to adult intelligence; it is also true (as mentioned above) that environment has, or can have, a strong effect on adult intelligence. The individual's genotype predisposes him or her toward a given IQ level, but various environmental factors can impede, or possibly even stimulate, the course of development of intelligence. For example, if humans are similar to the rats cited above, exposure to a highly stimulatory and interactive early post-natal environment may result in a higher IQ than exposure to a deficient environment. One can argue that every human child should be given a stimulating environment, and that those who do not have such stimulation are deprived. Others might view environmental stimulation as augmentation. Many of these are political points of view, however. It is logical to assume that, if society were to provide an optimal environment for all, the final differences in IQ would be solely the result of genetics.

As mentioned, if a genetic component to learning exists, it must have a corresponding biochemical expression. Therefore, learning must have some biochemical component. Attempts to study this aspect of learning were stimulated by the biochemical discoveries of protein synthesis in the 1960s. It became possible to study protein synthesis during the stages of learning. One of the first questions studied was whether new protein molecules were synthesized in the course of LTM consolidation.

Since messenger RNA must first be transcribed from DNA, one could assess the metabolic changes in each of these classes of molecules during LTM formation. DNA does not change during learning, which was expected to be the case, as new CNS cell growth can only be glial.

Studying RNA turnover was a much more difficult problem, made yet more difficult by the large amount of publicity surrounding experiments that seemed to indicate that RNA was a "learning molecule." Many poorly controlled and highly sensational experiments were performed that seemed to implicate RNA as fundamental to learning. There were even attempts to improve memory by feeding subjects RNA or its components. Eventually, carefully designed, well-controlled psychological experiments including specific inhibitors of transcription showed that new, specific RNA was synthesized during the learning of complex tasks. These tasks typically included both motor and cognitive aspects.

Similarly, carefully controlled, well-designed experiments with specific inhibitors of protein synthesis showed that new, specific protein molecules are made during LTM consolidation of complex motor and cognitive tasks. The nature of some of these molecules was determined at the University of North Carolina.

All lipids and carbohydrates are made by enzymes (proteins), as only nucleic acids and proteins are gene products. Post-translational changes in protein molecules, such as phosphorylation and glycosylation (i.e., attachment of sugars), are also effected by specific enzymes. Therefore, many biological molecules are the products of gene products and are determined by genes only indirectly. The above-mentioned investigations measured changes in several different kinds of molecules and found both phosphoproteins and glycoproteins to be prominent among the new substances specifically synthesized during LTM consolidation. These investigations also disclosed that a class of complex glycolipids, gangliosides, were being synthesized during LTM formation. All of these classes of molecules are concentrated in synapses. Therefore, new synaptic molecules of many kinds must be made during each acquisition of long-term learning. Since these molecules are not themselves direct gene products, but the products of interaction of gene products, many genes must be involved in determining the LTM formation process. Learning is therefore a *polygenic* characteristic (similar to height) in that it is strongly affected by the *interactions* of many genes, rather than being determined by a single gene or a small number of discrete genes. Further, gene interactions are more likely to be affected by environmental influences on the organism than the expressions of single genes. Therefore, the whole process is complex enough to include all the effects from both sides of the argument.

The fact that the new molecules synthesized during learning are synaptic molecules is strongly supportive of both the observation discussed above (that synaptic number is proportional to learning) and Hebb's synaptic network theory. It therefore seems reasonable to conclude that significant synaptic changes are occurring during learning and are a necessary part of that learning. After all of this work, the question of what specific synaptic changes are taking place remains. Although this question cannot yet be answered, speculation focuses on either changes that increase the size of pre-existing synapses or changes that make new ones. Supporting data indicate that both may occur. In fact, synapses may grow during learning. It may be that after a particular point is reached, further growth occurs by subdivision of existing synapses into multiple, smaller synapses.

Two further points need be made, about the role of STM consolidation into LTM and about the psychological state of the organism during learning. It has been known for many years that STM must be present for LTM to occur. If one waits too long to consolidate (or if a protein synthesis inhibitor is present), LTM is not formed. The information is forgotten, and acquiring the information requires complete relearning. Further studies of this phenomenon have shown that the converse is also true. Maintaining the presence of STM for longer periods of time increases the possibility of forming LTM from it.

A related issue, but more difficult to define and study, is the necessity for psychological "arousal." In practice, in learning experiments with rodents, arousal often means stress, or aversive arousal. Stimulatory drugs can also produce a state of arousal that enhances learning. These drugs, sometimes taken willingly by humans for their ability to produce pleasurable stimulation, have also been used in rodents to augment learning. Some kind of arousal state, either pleasurable or aversive, is therefore required for learning. A tranquil, unaroused rat does not make LTM.

As mentioned, the dopaminergic nigrostriatal system, which may be unconscious, may activate reflexive learning, and the noradrenergic locus ceruleus may activate the conscious learning system. In humans, the requirement for locus ceruleus activation of cognitive learning may translate into the necessity for motivation. One should not forget, however, that negative stimulation, i.e., stress, is also conducive to learning.

SPECIFIC SYNAPSES AND TRANSMITTERS

Indications regarding transmitter(s) specific for learning have come from studying mutants of *Drosophila*. Many years ago, Seymour Benzer developed a method for separating mutant fruit flies with learning problems from normal flies. The work is tedious, both the separation itself and the subsequent determination of whether the mutation was in the learning process or in other, related systems. (Fruit fly mutants with sensory deficiencies also learn more poorly.) Several mutations with specific learning deficiencies have been isolated, however. All have some kind of abnormality in their serotonergic synapses. Some of these mutants have abnormalities in other transmitter systems, as well, but defective serotonin function is the common feature.

The *Amnesiac* mutation learns normally, but forgets quickly. It has a decreased activity of dopa decarboxylase (i.e., aromatic amino acid decarboxylase), which is common to the synthetic pathways of several transmitters (Chapters 6 and 7). The *Turnip* mutation has poor initial learning, and at least one of its serotonin receptors has an increased K_D (i.e., it binds less well) for serotonin. The *Dunce* mutation also has poor initial learning and shows an increased level of cAMP. The *Rutabaga* mutation has poor initial learning and has a decreased level of cAMP. Since serotonin receptors are often associated with adenylyl cyclase in invertebrates, all of these mutants likely have modifications in their serotonergic systems. It is also fair to conclude that other transmitters besides serotonin, especially the catecholamines, may be involved, and that just the right levels of cAMP are necessary for normal learning.

Another invertebrate that has yielded much molecular information is *Aplysia*, the mollusk called the California sea hare. Kandel and Schwartz studied a sensory-motor link and have characterized a particular presynaptic synapse in detail. This system can be used to study both habituation and sensitization, as described earlier. Kandel and Schwartz showed that with habituation, less neurotransmitter is released with each successive repetition of a mild stimulus administered to the animal's skin. These investigators also showed that sensitization reversed this effect, causing an increase of transmitter release in response to a noxious stimulus to the head of the animal. This basic sensory-motor system connects sensory to motor neurons in a simple circuit (Figure 12-2). This simple network habituates with repetition, by decreased Ca^{++} mobilization in the synapses that activate the motor neurons. The mechanism is, in part, a time-lag delay, in which full recovery of Ca^{++} concentrations has not occurred by the time the next stimulus arrives.

The increased release of transmitter in sensitization is effected by a presynaptic synapse, coming from a neuron located near the animal's head (Figure 12-2). This neuron, by releasing its transmitter onto the presynaptic terminal innervating the motor neuron, is able to reverse habituation and cause an increased release of transmitter beyond that induced by the milder stimulus. The transmitter in this case, at the presynaptic synapse, is serotonin. The receptor, located in this case in the presynaptic terminal, is linked to adenylyl cyclase, and cAMP is elevated in this terminal as a result of the noxious stimulus. This system, possibly similar to that in the fruit flies, links learning to serotonin and cAMP.

Complete details of the mechanism of serotonin's production of sensitization in this system are not yet known, but some aspects of the mechanism have

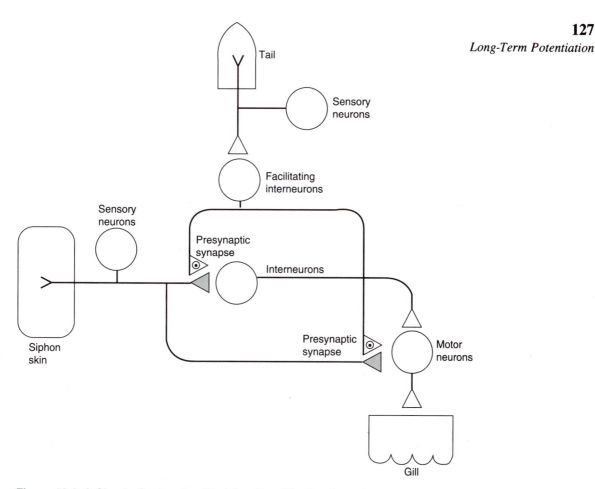

Figure 12-2 A Simple System for Studying Sensitization Learning

been worked out. As a result of the action of protein kinase A, stimulated by elevated cAMP, there is a decrease in the permeability of the plasma membrane to K^+. This decrease, in turn, prolongs presynaptic potentials in this synaptic terminal. Such a prolongation results in an increase in the total amount of calcium ion mobilized in the terminal, since K^+ permeability is the major mechanism for ending each presynaptic potential. The number of transmitter vesicles that are exocytosed into the synaptic cleft is directly proportional to the total amount of Ca^{++} mobilized. Finally, an increased number of vesicles produces an increased amount of transmitter released into the cleft. Therefore, the mechanism of learning (sensitization) in this case is the modification of a sensory-motor synapse by a third neuron's activation. This modification occurs presynaptically, thereby emphasizing the point that synapses are a major site of regulation within the CNS.

LONG-TERM POTENTIATION

Aplysia can be studied in vitro, but until relatively recently, learning in mammals could not be. It was discovered in the late 1970s that in vitro slices of rat hippocampus could produce a physiological change that might be related to learning in vivo. Such slices can be kept alive in vitro for many weeks, but are usually studied over a period of hours. Dr. Gary Lynch, and many others, observed that stimulating a particular pathway in the hippocampus with a particular frequency and intensity of electrical impulse would change the responsiveness of a group of neurons in the slice, and that this change was long-lasting. In fact, the modification lasted as long as the slice could be kept alive. Specific stimulating frequencies that produced a response potentiation were initially studied, and this phenomenon was called long-term potentiation, or LTP. Later, it was also found that a long-term inhibition, or depression (LTD), could be produced. One major initial question was whether this phenomenon could be shown to occur in vivo. It has since been shown, although not without controversy, that similar kinds of effects can be produced in the whole animal, by similar kinds of stimulation.

Detailed study of this phenomenon has been carried out over the past decade, because of its possible role in in vivo LTM formation. The research has indicated some specifics of the transmitter activity associated with development of LTP. The major focus has been on glutamate, with some additional evidence for the involvement of adenosine and possibly other amino acids. Glutamate's role in the hippocampus in LTP formation may involve all the excitatory amino acid receptors. Research on the NMDA receptors has been especially intense. NMDA receptor activation appears to be an essential part of LTP formation, and therefore NMDA receptors are implicated in the mechanism of learning in the whole organism.

Besides the study of the formation of LTP, work on its maintenance has also been ongoing. The phosphorylation of functional proteins in synapses is, not surprisingly, strongly implicated. Protein kinases, enzymes that increase the phosphorylation of such proteins, have been shown to have elevated activity during LTP formation and maintenance. Such a persistent elevation of enzyme function could result in a significant shift in the balance of phosphorylation–dephosphorylation of substrate proteins. If protein kinase activity is increased and the counterbalancing phosphatase activities are not, substrate proteins will be maintained in a more phosphorylated state. Since the level of phosphorylation is a major mechanism of regulation of protein activity, these data provide an outline, although one not yet totally filled in, of how learning might occur at the synaptic level.

SELF-STUDY QUESTIONS

Facts:

1. Define learning, STM, and LTM.

2. Describe the turnover of DNA, RNA, protein, and lipids during LTM consolidation.

3. Describe the anatomical areas necessary for LTM consolidation.

4. Describe the neurotransmitter and its synapse in the potentiation system of *Aplysia*.

Concepts:

1. Discuss the relationship between the number of synapses and IQ.

2. Discuss the roles of serotonin, norepinephrine, and psychological arousal in LTM formation.

3. Discuss the nature of the engram.

BIBLIOGRAPHY

Agranoff, B.W. 1989. Learning and memory. In *Basic Neurochemistry,* edited by G. Seigel, B. Agranoff, R.W. Albers, and P. Molinoff. New York: Raven Press.

Kandel, E.R. 1991. Cellular mechanisms of learning and the biological basis of individuality. In *Principles of Neural Science*, 3d ed., edited by E.R. Kandel, J.H. Schwartz, and T.M. Jessell. New York: Elsevier.

Kupferman, I. 1991. Learning and memory. In *Principles of Neural Science*, 3d ed., edited by E.R. Kandel, J.H. Schwartz, and T.M. Jessell. New York: Elsevier.

McEwen, B. 1989. Endocrine effects on the brain and their relationship to behavior. In *Basic Neurochemistry*, edited by G. Siegel, B. Agranoff, R.W. Albers, and P. Molinoff. New York: Raven Press.

Mishkin, M., Malamut, B., and Bachevalier, J. 1984. Memories and habits: Two neural systems. In *Neurobiology of Learning and Memory*, edited by G. Lynch, J.L. McGaugh, and N.M. Weinberger. New York: Guilford Press.

CHAPTER 13

Addiction and Receptor Regulation

INTRODUCTION

The term "addiction" is herein used in connection with drugs that affect the brain and, therefore, the mind. The World Health Organization (WHO) definition of addiction focuses on behavior: "A behavioral pattern of compulsive drug use, characterized by overwhelming involvement with the use of the drug, the securing of its supply, and a high tendency to relapse after withdrawal." Working definitions of addiction developed by people responsible for the care of addicts often focus on the impairment of life associated with drug use. A person may be addicted to a drug (for example, caffeine) but may be unimpaired by the drug. Because of the lack of impairment, neither society nor the addict's family and associates worry about the caffeine use. A similarly strong biological craving for a drug whose use is both illegal and incapacitating is quite a different matter. In that case a person is behaviorally involved with craving the drug to such an extent that it significantly damages his or her relationships at work and with family and friends. When the addict is deprived of the drug, a sickness occurs in response to the drug's absence. This sickness is called a withdrawal syndrome.

Each addictive drug produces its own characteristic withdrawal syndrome. The severity of the withdrawal syndrome varies with the drug, the level of addiction, and the duration of the addiction. The symptoms of the withdrawal syndrome often are opposite to those of the acute effects of the drug. For example, barbiturates have a depressant effect when used acutely, but withdrawal from chronic intake produces an extreme activation of many physiological systems, including the CNS. Affected individuals may experience seizures. In fact, sudden withdrawal from barbiturates can be lethal because of this overactivation. The withdrawal syndrome occurs because the organism's biochemical functioning has changed so as to incorporate the drug. This may be an attempt, by means of the kinds of biochemical regulatory mechanisms discussed earlier, to compensate for the drug's effects. As a result, repeated intake of the drug produces a smaller and smaller effect. In most cases, the drug user responds by increasing the dose in order to get the same experience felt previously. This effect, the need for a greater dose to produce the same result, is called **tolerance.** The accompanying effect, the derangement of the apparently "normal" functioning by removal of the drug, is called **dependence.** Although these two effects are not necessarily exactly the same, they normally occur together in a (biochemically) addicted individual. Tolerance and dependence are the classical signs of drug addiction.

If an acute dose of a drug clears the organism's body before another dose is taken, the onset of addiction is probably delayed. This is true of the biochemical development of dependence, tolerance, and addiction. ("Psychological" dependence occurs by a different mechanism.) If a subsequent drug dose is ingested before the last dose has been eliminated, the organism experiences a continuous exposure to the drug. With several addictive drugs, and especially with alcohol, this continuous drug level has been shown to be crucial for chemical dependence to develop. Experimental animals can develop ethanol dependence in fewer than one hundred hours if kept in an environment where ethanol is in the air they breathe. By this means a continuous, physiologically effective blood level of the drug is maintained in the animals, causing tolerance and dependence.

Biochemically, the addictive process can be thought of as the mechanism that produces the withdrawal syndrome. This is a long-term process by which chronic, steady-state levels of the drug become incorporated into the person's "normal" biology. Without the drug, the addict experiences a sickness that results from its absence. This long-term process typically takes place in days to weeks or longer. This places the addiction process on a time scale similar to that of long-term memory consolidation—i.e., the time required to replace proteins in the synapse (since the proteins must be synthesized in the cell body and transported to the terminal).

Given the timing, the addiction process likely requires changes in genetic expression, i.e., changes in the regulation of synthesis of proteins and nucleic acids. Therefore, the development of an addiction to a drug is a highly complex process, involving many levels of regulation and bearing some similarity to types of learning. Chapter 12 discussed a distinction between reflexive and cognitive (declarative) learning. Reflexive learning (e.g., the formation of a habit) is incorporated into the brain by a significantly different physiological system than is cognitive (higher) learning. Both types of learning share the fact that something new is being recorded in the CNS, and that it becomes easier to recall or repeat the new activity after the learning has occurred. Addiction to a particular drug may involve either the reflexive or the declarative system at its onset. As the time scale is somewhat longer than usually required for cognitive learning, addiction may be more analogous to habit formation or reflexive learning. Indeed, this process has many features in common with habituation (see Chapter 12). (Indeed, many addicts refer to their drug-related behavior as a "habit.") In the development of addiction, as in habituation, the effect of the stimulus (drug) decreases with multiple repetitions and, after sufficient time, results in major structural changes in the affected synapses.

An additional point worth noting in this context is that the addiction process is distinct from the mental effects of the drug, which are presumably the reason the drug is used in the first place. Therefore, in trying to understand addiction to any particular drug, one must understand both the drug's effect on the central nervous system and the biochemical responses that result in tolerance and dependence.

At the most fundamental level, addiction may be thought of as an example of receptor regulation. In this context, the word "receptor" may have a somewhat different meaning from that used in the discussion of transmitters. The receptor(s) for a drug are the molecules or classes of molecules that interact with the drug and produce the body's biological responses to it. Some addictive drugs, such as opiates, may have their most important effects on the receptors for a specific group of transmitters (e.g., mu receptors). Other drugs, such as alcohol, while having important effects on the receptors of some transmitters, also affect other brain structures, such as membranes. These membrane effects, produced by the physical chemistry of the molecule rather than by specific binding properties, may be an important part of alcohol's effects. Membranes might therefore be considered as part of alcohol's receptors, by the above definition. Cocaine has, among other properties, a major effect on catecholamine transport, and barbiturates, among other actions, inhibit oxidative phosphorylation. Thus, the receptive portions of the CNS for addictive drugs involve some transmitters' receptors but also include other functional structures.

Additionally, it has been shown in recent years that genetics plays an important role in many drug addictions. The largest of these studies have used adoption records of several thousand people in Scandinavian countries. A genetic predisposition has been most clearly shown for alcohol and opiates, but a similar biological predisposition may exist for other drugs, as well. In the light of all of this, in order to understand addiction to even a single drug, it is necessary to understand the details of the mechanism of the drug's acute effects, the mechanism of its chronic effects (i.e., the addictive process), and the basis of the biological predisposition. Since each addictive drug's mechanism of action may be different from those of other drugs, its chronic effects and the basis of the predisposition for its use may also be unique.

The study of addiction is further complicated by the fact that most important drugs of addiction affect every cell in the body in some way, although the focus of addiction research is generally on the CNS. This is because people presumably consume addictive drugs for the effects produced on the brain and mind. Thus, each drug is the focus of a separate biochemical and medical study. The present discussion can only be a brief introduction to the topic.

MECHANISMS OF ADDICTION

The drive for the achievement of homeostasis is the most common form of response to chronic change occurring in biological systems and may be the primary mechanism underlying the addiction process. Long-term changes that compensate for the acute drug effects imply that homeostatic mechanisms are involved. For example, opiates acutely inhibit the locus ceruleus (LC). Crystals of an opiate, chronically implanted near the LC, initially inhibit it, but the baseline activity of the LC eventually returns toward normal despite the continuing presence of the drug. When this happens, it indicates that the drug's presence has been (partially) compensated for by regulatory changes in LC activity. If the crystal is removed at this point, the LC shows a marked increase in baseline activity. This increased activity, possibly related to a phenomenon resembling a withdrawal syndrome, is in the opposite direction from the acute, inhibitory effect of the drug. Homeostatic regulatory mechanisms, in this case, have apparently responded to the drug's inhibitory effect by restoring activity toward normal (i.e., the pre-drug baseline) levels even in the drug's presence. This process involves the development of a resistance to the drug's acute effects and leads to tolerance and dependence.

In the presence of this homeostatic compensation, a higher dose of the drug is required to produce the same degree of acute inhibition. This may be the basis of tolerance, in this case achieved by a compensatory increase in endogenous LC activity. During the period of tolerance, there would be increased activity of the LC if the drug were removed. This increased activity may be the basis of the withdrawal syndrome, and therefore may be the mechanism of dependence. Some such type of homeostatic chemical compensation may be the basis of many addictions.

TYPES OF ADDICTION

The drugs that are the most common cause of addiction are also those that have been most heavily studied: (1) alcohol, barbiturates, and tranquilizers; (2) cocaine and amphetamines; and (3) opiates. The members of the first group are known to interact with the GABA-A receptor and other structures, and are depressants. Those in the second group are excitatory to the organism and are known to act in the synapses of catecholamine neurotransmitters. The opiates are depressants and are agonists for enkephalin, endorphin, and dynorphin receptors.

Each drug has specific acute CNS effects, which can be studied independently from the addiction process. Each drug also has effects in other tissues if taken chronically, producing addiction. These can be studied separately. For each of these groups the role of genetic susceptibility and the kind of mechanism that might produce a predisposition for its use are only subjects of speculation at this time.

ALCOHOL

Ethyl alcohol (ethanol) may be mankind's oldest addictive psychotropic drug. It is still probably the most widely used and may be the drug to which the largest number of people are addicted. Alcohol has been shown to produce manifold effects. Every cell in the body is affected to some degree. The most serious biological consequences of chronic alcohol consumption can be divided into two broad categories: metabolic effects in the liver and molecular and cellular effects in the brain. Both categories include acute and chronic components.

Research on the biochemistry of alcohol addiction has focused not only on neurotransmitter receptor regulation but also on metabolic pathways, membrane transport, and membrane structure. In recent years, a focus on ethanol's effects on the GABA-A receptor has appeared. Because of the numerous effects of ethanol, however, it is difficult to conclude which is most important in determining the causes of the addictive disease called alcoholism.

The Effects of Ethanol

It was established as early as the 1940s that ethanol inhibits the oxygen consumption of brain cells in vitro in an unusual way. Isolated brain cells have two different levels of metabolism, "resting," when the cell is not firing, and "active," when it is generating action potentials. The active metabolism is superimposed on the resting metabolism. Resting oxygen consumption is more than half (about 60 percent) of the total. Ethanol specifically inhibits the active metabolism, an effect shared by other organic alcohols of the same family, e.g., methanol, propanol, butanol, etc.

Homogenized cells, i.e., those without an intact plasma membrane, cannot fire, and this inhibition does not occur. Part of the research on ethanol's effects on the CNS continues to focus on these membrane actions, which may not involve a particular, individual receptor molecule. This inhibition is apparently produced by the physical chemical properties of ethanol in membranes, rather than by any specific binding property.

Ethanol produces an acute "disordering" effect on membranes. Chronic ethanol exposure, however, results in membranes' becoming more "ordered." Changes in membrane lipid composition, that of phosphatidyl inositols (PI) in particular, appear to be of greatest significance in this regard. This inference is based on measurements of membrane lipid fractions from the brains of rats chronically exposed to alcohol and compared to those of untreated animals. In such experiments, only the PI fraction from the chronic ethanol-treated animals produced the "ordering" effect when added to the membrane extracts from control animals.

Ethanol also affects the GABA-A receptor. It is an allosteric activator, although it does not act in the same way as GABA. The GABA-A receptor has allosteric binding sites distinct from those that bind the transmitter. These secondary sites, present at a different subunit location from the GABA binding sites, modify the binding of GABA to its sites on the receptor. The secondary, alcohol-sensitive, sites have an indirect effect on GABA–receptor interaction, increasing the GABA effect. Similar secondary GABA receptor effects are shown by benzodiazepines, alcohols, and barbiturates. This secondary site is the normal binding site of an endogenous peptide (Chapter 9).

There is further evidence that a subclass of GABA-A receptors has a specific affinity for ethanol and that this subclass may be most affected by it. A large concentration of this subclass of GABA receptors exists in the cerebellum, where their affinity for ethanol may be part of the mechanism of alcohol-induced ataxia (disorder of walking). The ataxia that alcohol-intoxicated persons experience may in part be explained by the interaction between this subunit of the GABA-A receptor and ethanol. It is possible that this subunit is not found in equal amounts in all people, and therefore it could be a part of the genetic susceptibility to alcohol's effects.

In addition to its specific activation of the GABA-A receptor and its generalized effects on the plasma membranes of neurons, ethanol also produces a specific inhibition of the locus ceruleus (Chapter 6). This is similar to what is believed to be the major effect of opiates, and a significant part of the depressant action of ethanol may come from this activity.

Finally, these membrane actions are in contrast to alcohol's effects on liver and other tissues. In the latter locations, metabolism of alcohol produces an imbalance in the coenzymes of oxidation–reduction, and this imbalance leads to much of the resulting tissue damage. Specifically, ethanol raises the $NADH/NAD^+$ ratio. Since ethanol is poorly metabolized in the brain, its effects in this organ are most likely due to other phenomena, e.g., membrane and receptor interactions.

Ethanol Addiction

Ethanol depresses neuronal metabolism acutely. The addicted state may involve compensation for the chronic presence of alcohol aimed at restoring a more appropriate metabolic level. The withdrawal syndrome from chronic ethanol (i.e., delirium tremens, or the "DTs") is a hyperactivation of the organism. This indicates a possible homeostatic mechanism for this addiction process. These compensatory, long-term changes could occur in the chemical properties of plasma membranes, including both changes in membrane composition and changes in the number of GABA-A receptors.

The above-mentioned membrane and receptor properties of ethanol are a significant part of the CNS effects of ethanol. The metabolic properties of ethanol also must be considered in attempting to understand ethanol's long-term effects on the body. The liver is the most important of the other organs affected by alcohol, as it is the major site of ethanol metabolism and thus the site of its most important metabolic effects. In addition to the regulatory and degenerative changes that have been induced in their nervous systems, chronic alcoholics may suffer long-term destructive changes in their livers.

Ethanol is metabolized to CO_2 and H_2O by the liver and other tissues, producing energy. The complete catabolism of one molecule of ethanol requires both the cytoplasmic and mitochondrial compartments in the cell, as does the metabolism of carbohydrates. However, ethanol appears to produce pathological effects in both compartments. That is, although ethanol itself may be fully catabolized within the liver, its presence in significant quantity causes metabolic imbalances that affect the metabolism of other substrates.

The first step of ethanol metabolism is an oxidation. Alcohol dehydrogenase is the cytoplasmic enzyme that oxidizes ethanol to acetaldehyde while simultaneously reducing NAD^+ to NADH. Aldehydes in general are toxic; acetaldehyde is no exception. The aldehyde is quickly removed by oxidation to acetic acid under normal circumstances. This oxidation is accomplished by an aldehyde dehydrogenase or by an aldehyde oxidase. It is not entirely clear whether this second step occurs in cytoplasm or in mitochondria, although a consensus now seems to favor mitochondria.

The first step occurs in the cytoplasm, the results of which can be harmful, especially if the alcohol consumption occurred in the fasting state (i.e., in the absence of other substrates for liver metabolism). The primary mechanism for the harmful effects is the shift in the $NAD^+/NADH$ ratio. In normal cytoplasm, this ratio favors NAD^+, being in the range of several hundred to a thousand. Reduction of a significant fraction of NAD^+ to NADH changes the ratio greatly, which in turn affects many other cellular pathways. Two of the most important processes affected are those that cause fatty liver and hypoglycemia.

It has been known for many years that high alcohol consumption causes a fatty liver, acutely and chronically. A night of heavy drinking leads to a fatty liver the next morning. There are many possible mechanisms for this effect. For example, the fact that ethanol increases cytoplasmic NADH has been suggested as causing a rise in fatty acid synthesis. This particular mechanism, although not impossible, should be considered unlikely, in part because NADH is not involved in fatty acid synthesis. Two other mechanisms for the production of fatty liver are plausible, however: inhibition of protein synthesis and inhibition of fatty acid oxidation. Direct measurements on liver cells in the presence of alcohol have not shown large increases in fatty acid synthesis, but have shown a significant inhibition of fatty acid oxidation. The mechanism for this effect is not entirely understood but may be due to an inhibition by cytoplasmic NADH of the transport mechanisms that fatty acids use to enter mitochondria. Clearly, fat accumulation in the liver could be due to decreased catabolism as well as to increased synthesis.

Ethanol has also been shown to inhibit protein synthesis in doses comparable to those achieved in vivo. This effect of ethanol, in fact, was observed during the earliest experiments on protein synthesis. Contemporary researchers independently demonstrated that inhibiting protein synthesis resulted in a fatty liver. The mechanism of this appears to be in the liver's synthesis of blood lipoproteins. These complex molecules contain large amounts of both fat and protein. If the synthesis of the protein portion of the molecules is impaired, the fats cannot be released from the tissue and therefore build up within it.

Ethanol also has an important effect on glucose metabolism. In the fasting state (i.e., several hours after a meal containing carbohydrate), the liver synthesizes much of the blood glucose by the pathway known as gluconeogenesis. One of the reactions of gluconeogenesis, the conversion of malate to oxaloacetate, must occur in the cytoplasm of the hepatocyte. In order for this reaction to proceed in the appropriate direction, the cytoplasm must have a high NAD^+/NADH ratio (Figure 13-1). When alcohol is consumed in the fasting state, this ratio is diminished, and the reaction is inhibited. In this situation, gluconeogenesis cannot occur, and the resulting hypoglycemia can be life-threatening, by producing a coma. Misdiagnosis of hypoglycemic coma can result in permanent brain damage. If blood glucose falls below about 1 mM, the brain is deprived of one of its two essential substrates, and coma often results. If the condition persists for many hours, neuronal death and subsequent brain damage can occur (see Chapter 14).

In addition to inhibiting gluconeogenesis, fasting ethanol consumption leads to an increase in lactic acid (lactate) production by the liver. The increased NADH produces lactate from pyruvate. This increase in lactate also has pathological consequences. Lactate is a metabolic dead end; it can only be converted back to pyruvate or excreted from the body. Blood lactate is normally taken up either by the liver, as a substrate for gluconeogenesis, or by the heart, for energy production. If the liver cannot use lactate for glucose synthesis, much of the lactate remains in the blood. The excess, beyond what the heart can consume, contributes to **acidosis.**

Additionally, lactate excretion by the kidneys requires the use of anion transporters, and excessive blood lactate therefore inhibits the urinary excretion of other anions. This is one mechanism by which fasting alcohol consumption can bring on an attack of gout (or gouty arthritis). The uric acid formed in blood from purines must be excreted, as the body cannot metabolize uric acid further. As increased blood lactate interferes with the excretion of uric acid, uric acid's concentration in blood rises, and it is therefore more likely to precipitate in joints and cause an acute attack of gout. This occurs because the normal level of uric acid in blood, in men predisposed to gout, is not much below its maximum solubility. The solubility is actually exceeded in some people with a genetic predisposition to the disease.

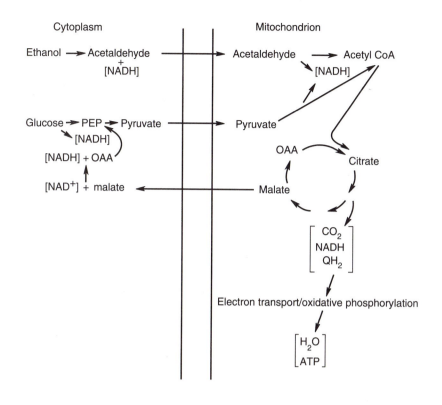

Cytoplasm   Mitochondrion

Ethanol → Acetaldehyde ────────→ Acetaldehyde ──→ Acetyl CoA
              +   [NADH]
           [NADH]

Glucose → PEP → Pyruvate ────────→ Pyruvate
           [NADH]
                                          OAA
[NADH] + OAA   Citrate

[NAD⁺] + malate ←──────────── Malate

                                        ⎡ CO₂ ⎤
                                        ⎢ NADH ⎥
                                        ⎣ QH₂ ⎦

                  Electron transport/oxidative phosphorylation

                                        ⎡ H₂O ⎤
                                        ⎣ ATP ⎦

Figure 13-1 The Compartmentation of the Metabolism of Ethanol and Glucose

Thus, alcohol has toxic effects on both brain and liver (as well as other organs, such as kidneys and joints), and those toxicities occur by distinct mechanisms. Alcohol is not metabolized in large quantities in the brain but produces physical and chemical membrane and receptor effects. The liver, which does metabolize alcohol, experiences toxic effects from this metabolism, and especially from the excessive NADH levels produced in cytoplasm.

The chronic effects in both organs involve compensations for the effects of ethanol. There may be changes in GABA-A receptor number or in the sensitivity of the receptors to ethanol's effects. Either could explain tolerance and dependence. The liver responds to chronic ethanol intake with less fatty buildup, but some people continue to increase their ethanol intake to the point that their livers may no longer be able to compensate. Many long-term alcoholics may develop a chronic fatty liver, proceeding to an alcoholic **hepatitis,** and, eventually, to **cirrhosis.** This liver toxicity may not be part of the primary addiction process, but a pathological side effect of chronic high ethanol consumption.

None of the above, however, addresses the question of predisposition to alcoholism. Adoption studies in Scandinavian countries have shown, to the satisfaction of most observers, that there is a significant genetic susceptibility to the development of alcoholism. Genetics is not the only factor, of course, as the availability of and willingness to use alcohol are essential for the disease process to occur. There is still no clear indication of what the predisposing factor might be. Theoretically, it could involve membrane lipid structure, the structure or number of GABA-A receptors, the endogenous arousal or activation of the locus ceruleus, or other factors. This is a fertile area of future research.

BENZODIAZEPINES AND BARBITURATES

The benzodiazepines (BZPs), which are among the most widely prescribed drugs, work as secondary allosteric effectors of the GABA-A receptor (Chapter 9). Their tranquilizing effects probably derive primarily from their ability to increase the effects of GABA. Therefore, the development of an addiction to BZPs probably involves molecular changes in the GABA-A receptors. Either decreased synthesis of GABA-A receptors, which would then require a larger amount of GABA (and/or BZP) to be effective, or a change in the binding characteristics of the receptors could explain tolerance and dependence. Other mechanisms are also possible.

In addition to acting as secondary allosteric effectors of the GABA-A receptor, barbiturates, like ethanol, have other effects as well. Barbiturates inhibit oxidative metabolism, especially at the level of the mitochondrion. The first electron transport complex (often called complex I, or NADH-coenzyme Q reductase, or NADH reductase) has been known for many years to be inhibited by barbiturates. Again, like ethanol, this inhibitory action of barbiturates affects nearly every cell in the body. Molecular changes in response to chronic barbiturate consumption are homeostatic in nature, at least as judged by the associated withdrawal syndrome. Withdrawal from barbiturates often includes a hyperexcitation of many organs, including the CNS. This hyperexcitation can be so extreme as to result in death. Given the extreme nature of the withdrawal syndrome, changes in the function or the number of mitochondria might be involved in barbiturate addiction.

COCAINE AND AMPHETAMINES

The acute effects of cocaine and amphetamines are predominantly excitatory in nature; the drugs produce a feeling of greater energy and greater psychological arousal. These effects are usually coupled with diminished appetite and need for sleep, all of which support the organism's increased state of readiness. The effects are in the opposite direction from those of most other addictive drugs, which are depressants, or "downers," and which decrease the organism's state of readiness. Therefore, one might expect at least the mechanisms of the acute effects and the nature of the biological predisposition to using the drugs to be quite different from other drugs.

Both cocaine and the amphetamines appear to have their acute actions focused primarily in catecholaminergic synapses (Chapter 6). Since catecholamines are mostly excitatory to the organism, these drugs would be expected to increase the activity of catecholaminergic synapses. Cocaine, for example, while affecting many functional molecules in the synapses of several different transmitters, may produce a major part of its psychological effects by inhibiting the uptake of catecholamines from their synaptic clefts. Such an effect would increase the action of the transmitter by keeping it in the cleft longer, confirming the above-mentioned expectation about its mechanism of action. This action does not appear to be a direct competitive inhibition of the re-uptake transporter, but seems instead to be an allosteric inhibition, which is more indirect.

Amphetamines' mechanism of action is even more complex than that of cocaine, since amphetamines appear to interact at most of the possible sites of intervention in catecholaminergic synapses. Some of the actions increase synaptic activity and some decrease it, but the overall, net effect is stimulation of the organism. Therefore, an increase in synaptic activity is expected. Thus, the two drugs are similar in that they produce similar changes in the psychological and behavioral state of the organism. In fact, amphetamines and cocaine cross-react in many of their effects. It is also worth noting that both drugs appear to stimulate some of the same neural structures (such as the locus ceruleus) that are inhibited by many addictive depressant drugs.

Although the mechanisms of the long-term regulatory changes that are responsible for the development of addiction may be similar for all drugs, the specific molecules being affected in cocaine and amphetamine addiction are likely quite different from those affected in other addictions. For example, if addiction to cocaine were to involve an increased number (or a decreased sensitivity) of re-uptake transporters for dopamine and/or noradrenaline, the resulting effects on the organism's behavior would be quite different from—in fact, opposite to— those of addiction to benzodiazepines or alcohol. The addicted state, in which these long-term changes have been made, would result in decreased activity at catecholamine synapses in the absence of the drug. This would put the addicted person on a chronic "downer" (unless more drug were consumed) that might be expected to be associated with depression. In fact, depression and increased sleep and fatigue are characteristic of people who withdraw from chronic, heavy use of either drug.

The above observations provide further support to the homeostatic theory of biochemical addiction, but are highly oversimplified. In fact, the organism does not develop tolerance to some of the acute effects of cocaine and amphetamines, and may even become more sensitive to some of these effects with chronic use. The higher mental functions are especially affected in this way, with large doses of these drugs producing a psychosis-like state, even in chronic, heavy users. The mechanism of these effects and the role they play in the abuse of these drugs are currently unknown, and are subjects of considerable research.

OPIATES

The opium poppy's special abilities to relieve pain have been utilized beneficially for at least a century. The endogenous brain compounds that also activate opiate receptors were discovered only within the last twenty years. The structures of the endogenous molecules are markedly distinct from the opiate alkaloids produced in plants (see Chapter 8). Endogenous opiates are all peptides, and they come from at least three distinct precursors, making three different families of transmitters. Despite the amount of information gained in the last few years about opiate receptors and their mechanisms of action, it is still not clear why some people are more strongly attracted than others to the alkaloid opiate receptor agonists. Whatever the reason, certain people are at greater risk than normal of becoming addicted to opioids. The existence of such a predisposition has been suspected for years, based on both adoption studies and observation of opiate use in populations. The latter indicate that not all people are equally attracted to opiates, even when they are made universally available. In fact, studies in different parts of the world have indicated that about 10 percent of a human population are at greatest risk for opiate addiction. The basis of this predisposition is a subject for future research.

The major acute effect of exogenous opiates is tranquilization, but it is not the same state produced by ethanol, barbiturates, or the benzodiazepines. One possible mechanism of action has been discussed in Chapter 8, that of inhibiting the release of substance P, the pain transmitter, from its terminals. This action of opiates helps explain their analgesic properties and, therefore, much of their medical utility. Although it is theoretically possible to explain part of the opiate addiction phenomenon by the desire for pain relief, this theory probably does not fully explain such addiction.

Agonists for opiate receptors also inhibit many neurons and in several locations in the brain. One important inhibitory site is the locus ceruleus (LC), mentioned before as the main location of noradrenergic cell bodies in the brain. One can produce opiate addiction in an animal experimentally by implanting a small crystal of the drug close to the LC. Since the LC is known to be both a source of psychological arousal and a pleasure center, the effects of opiates on this nucleus could be a major part of the incentive for taking the drugs and of the mechanism of development of tolerance and dependence.

CONCLUSION

All of the addictive drugs mentioned in this chapter, both stimulatory and depressant, have effects on one or more of the pleasure centers (see Chapter 6). Cocaine and amphetamines affect both DA and NE synapses, increasing the catecholamine's effects. Opiates inhibit many neurons, certainly both dopaminergic cells and the neurons of the LC. GABA also inhibits many neurons, including those in the LC. Ethanol has also been shown to produce a relatively specific inhibition of LC neurons. Given the importance to an organism of the pleasure/pain balance and the effectiveness of these drugs at altering this balance, it is not surprising that drugs that interfere in this system would be abused. Many people will seek to alter the endogenous pleasure/pain balance by exogenous means. A greater understanding of the mechanisms involved with each drug, and in each patient, may allow the development of effective, individualized interventions.

As mentioned, the use of, and addiction to, each different drug presents a separate biochemical research problem, and each of these can be grouped under three different general questions: What are the mechanisms of the acute effects of the drug? What are the mechanisms of the chronic response (i.e., addiction development)? What are the predisposing factors?

As we have seen, the chemical mechanisms of a drug's acute effects vary with the drug, but most addictive drugs interact with some neurotransmitters' receptors. Depressants often interact with GABA receptors, and stimulatory drugs often affect catecholamines. Besides receptors, many drugs affect other functional parts of cells, such as the plasma membrane (ethanol) or the inner mitochondrial membrane (barbiturates). For each drug, the effect on the organism is the sum, or the resultant, of all these individual effects taken together. Working out the details of each of these actions and determining the relative importance of each will require a great deal more research.

The development of addiction (and tolerance) in response to chronic, heavy use of a drug requires long-term changes in the chemistry of the brain. Each drug has a different profile of effects, but similar mechanisms might operate in the addictive process. As we have seen, the most common kinds of long-term changes are in the homeostatic direction, more like habituation than like higher learning. The brain attempts to compensate for the presence of the drug by diminishing its effects and incorporating it into the ongoing, dynamic cellular activity. These kinds of changes cause the withdrawal syndrome to have the opposite characteristics of the acute effects of the drug. With any drug, these chronic changes require modifications in the level of synthesis of important brain macromolecules. Thus, major changes in the rate of synthesis of RNA and protein molecules are necessary for addiction to develop. (For example, one set of experiments indicated that inhibiting all protein synthesis in the brain prevents addiction to opiates.)

Little is yet known about the factors that predispose people to addiction to particular drugs, although there is evidence that such predispositions exist. It is also clear that a predisposition to use a drug is not the only factor in addiction. The predisposition is certainly not sufficient to cause addiction; it also is not necessary, as addiction can be created in experimental animals. But discovering the nature of the predisposition could be enormously helpful in counseling patients and greatly useful to a recovering person trying to plan his or her own life.

As indicated earlier, at the moment much of the speculation regarding predisposition focuses on the locus ceruleus (LC). Its role as a pleasure center, however ambiguous that role might be (Chapter 6), and its role in setting psychological arousal make it a likely suspect for being involved in drug abuse. The fact that all major addictive drugs have some effect, either inhibitory or stimulatory, on the LC supports this concept. Other transmitters, and other brain pleasure centers, may also be involved, particularly the mesolimbic, mesocortical dopaminergic system (Chapter 6). Drugs such as cocaine that affect both catecholamine systems are extremely attractive to many organisms, including many people. (Cocaine is the most strongly reinforcing molecule in lower mammals yet discovered.) Therefore, it is possible, even likely, that people seek to have greater control over the activity of their pleasure centers, and many turn to drugs that alter that activity.

SELF-STUDY QUESTIONS

Facts:

1. Define addiction, tolerance, and dependence.

2. What structures do each of the drugs discussed (ethanol, BZPs, barbiturates, cocaine, amphetamines, and opiates) affect most prominently?

3. Which neurotransmitters are most likely to be involved in the development of drug addiction?

Concepts:

1. Describe the likely role of membrane fluidity in ethanol addiction.

2. Describe the likely role of the LC in drug addiction.

3. Discuss possible mechanisms for a genetic predisposition to the use of molecules that are exogenous to the human body.

4. Discuss homeostatic regulatory mechanisms and how these could lead to tolerance and dependence.

5. Discuss the relationship between drug addiction and learning.

BIBLIOGRAPHY

Gilman, A.G., Goodman, L.S., Rall, T.N., and Murad, F. 1990. *The Pharmacological Basis of Therapeutics*, 8th ed. New York: Pergamon Press.

Hemmings, G., ed. 1980. *Biochemistry of Schizophrenia and Addiction*. Baltimore, MD: University Park Press.

Lieber, C.S. 1988. Biochemical and molecular basis of alcohol-induced injury to liver and other tissues. *New England Journal of Medicine* 319: 1639–1650.

Mitchell, M.C., and Herlong, H.F. 1986. Alcohol and nutrition: Caloric value, bioenergetics, and relationship to liver damage. *Annual Review of Nutrition* 6: 457–474.

Pickens, R.W., and Svikis, D.S. 1988. Biological vulnerability to drug abuse. NIDA Research Monograph 89. Washington, DC: U.S. Dept. of Health and Human Services.

Wise, R.A., and Rompre, P.P. 1989. Brain dopamine and reward. *Ann. Rev. Psychol.* 40: 191–225.

CHAPTER 14

Brain Energy Metabolism

OVERVIEW

Because it is so closely associated with mental function, the overall metabolism of brain is one of the most interesting and important aspects of neurobiology. As brain metabolism changes, so does mentation, with the degree of change in either reflected directly in the other. This overall correlation of mind and metabolism has been known for generations, but the details are still not well enough established to characterize it completely. Some details of brain metabolism have become clear in recent years, however.

One of the first peculiarities of brain metabolism is that it is heavily based on a single organic substrate, glucose. There are other substrates that can be used, but in the normal, healthy, adult human brain, glucose is the only substrate significantly catabolized for energy production. This fact, coupled with the fact that the brain has an unusually high level of metabolism (about 20 percent of the body's total oxygen consumption takes place in a tissue that has about 2 percent of the body's mass), means that the glucose turnover in blood is predominantly for the brain's use. There are a few other tissues that also use glucose nearly exclusively, such as the testes. There are also situations, such as during heavy exercise, in which muscle tissue will use large amounts of blood glucose. But under ordinary, resting circumstances, the brain uses most of the glucose cleared from blood. Because of this, the physiology of glucose uptake by the brain is quite important to brain metabolism, although it is also still not completely understood.

In addition to a continuous supply of glucose, the normal brain also requires a continuous oxygen supply. The oxidation of glucose accounts for essentially 100 percent of brain energy production. A disruption of the continuous supply of either substrate for any significant length of time will result in loss of brain function (i.e., consciousness). If the interruption continues, brain cell death results.

In addition to a continuous supply of substrates, the brain must also deal with the products of glucose's metabolism, carbon dioxide and water. The disposal of water is not thought to be a serious problem, although brain **edema** can have serious clinical consequences. Normal CNS tissue, however, must dispose of unusually large amounts of CO_2, which result from the catabolism of glucose. Since CO_2 is the acidic component of the primary acid/base buffer in the body, this CO_2 must be removed rapidly in order to prevent acidosis.

143

A measurement used to study overall metabolic balance in any tissue is the respiratory quotient (RQ), defined as the number of moles of CO_2 produced divided by the number of moles of O_2 consumed. This ratio can be applied to a cell, an organ, an organism, or an individual reaction sequence. The RQ varies depending on the substrate(s) used. Energy substrates require different amounts of oxygen for complete catabolism, depending on their relative state of oxidation prior to use. For example, fatty acids, which are fully metabolized in vivo to CO_2 and water, yield an RQ of about 0.7. That is, it takes more than one oxygen molecule to produce a molecule of carbon dioxide. Simple carbohydrates, such as glucose, are also completely catabolized to CO_2 and water, with an RQ of 1.0. That is, carbohydrate combustion requires exactly one mole of oxygen for each mole of carbon dioxide produced.

The RQ for the brain is commonly measured, both for the information it can provide and because it is relatively easy to gain access to blood flowing exclusively from the brain, in the jugular vein. In fact, RQ is easier to measure in humans than in most experimental animals, because of the anatomy of the jugular vein. In order to calculate RQ, it is necessary to measure the A-V differences (arterial concentration minus venous concentration) of CO_2 and O_2 across the brain. A sample of arterial blood from any site will suffice, as arterial blood circulates so quickly that it is equivalent throughout the body. The jugular vein is easily accessed in humans, and it contains about 97 percent cerebral venous blood as it exits the cranium. Therefore, by measuring the arteriovenous (A-V) differences across the brain for carbon dioxide (negative) and oxygen (positive), one can calculate the molar ratio (RQ). It is typically between 0.97 and 1.03. An RQ between these levels indicates that only carbohydrate is being oxidized in sufficient quantity to provide adequate ATP for brain work.

It is possible for the RQ to be higher than 1.0 in situations in which metabolic oxidations occur without the consumption of oxygen. A common example of such a situation is the activation of the pentose phosphate "shunt," which produces CO_2 without consuming oxygen. Cells that are using the pentose phosphate pathway in combination with other metabolic pathways may have RQs much higher than 1.0. This situation most commonly occurs when the tissue has a need for fat synthesis (the pentose phosphate shunt is necessary to produce cofactors for synthesizing fatty acids). Therefore, an RQ significantly above 1.0 may be found in the CNS of growing children. The brain and spinal cord contain large amounts of fat, most of which is synthesized in the first few years after birth. Fat catabolism produces the lowest RQ (0.7), and fat synthesis produces the highest. Therefore, the RQ in the brain theoretically ranges from 0.7 to greater than 1.0.

Ketone bodies, released into blood from liver during starvation or a high fat intake, can also be used by brain. Acetoacetate (one of the ketone bodies) also has an RQ of 1.0 and can also be metabolized in the brain. However, when ketone bodies are released from the liver, acetoacetate is present in equilibrium with beta-hydroxybutyrate, and both are released. Both substrates can be catabolized in the brain. Beta-hydroxybutyrate predominates in the equilibrium, with a ratio of about 3:1. As beta-hydroxybutyrate has an RQ of 0.89, the RQ for the mixture is about 0.93. Additionally, the brain cannot use ketone bodies exclusively. A maximum of about 60 percent of total brain metabolism can be derived from ketone bodies; the remainder must be supplied by glucose. This is true under even the most extreme conditions (e.g., fasting for several months). Therefore, brain

RQ with maximum ketone body catabolism is about 0.95. This is lower than what is usually found but is still not far from 1.0.

If brain nutrition is compromised, however, the RQ can fall significantly. For example, RQs as low as 0.85 have been measured in elderly patients with atherosclerosis. Only a few explanations for such a low RQ are possible. The energy substrates that yield RQs this low (i.e., fats and/or amino acids) do not cross the blood–brain barrier in adequate quantities to affect CNS energy metabolism significantly. If the barrier is modified in these patients, it is likely to be less permeable than normal, because of the thickened blood vessel walls. Therefore, significant amounts of proteins (i.e., amino acids) and/or fats must be being catabolized and used as substrates for oxidative metabolism *within* brain cells. The inference from such observations is that endogenous brain molecules are being catabolized—that is, brain substance is being broken down. This is obviously to the long-term detriment of brain function.

Consumption of ketone bodies in the brain was initially shown to occur during prolonged fasting. Many have concluded from this that the brain "adapts" to the chronic presence of ketone bodies in blood, becoming able to oxidize them for energy. However, L. Sokoloff has shown that this is not the case in the brain, although other tissues may so adapt. During infancy, the brain contains high levels of the two special enzymes necessary for ketone body consumption. One of these enzymes converts beta-hydroxybutyrate to acetoacetate, and the other enables acetoacetate to enter the citric acid cycle. This high capacity for ketone body metabolism in infants is apparently related to the high levels of ketone bodies in blood, which are in turn due to the high fat content of milk. As mammals mature, the brain levels of these two enzymes diminish. This change occurs around the time of weaning and the concomitant change of diet. The brains of adult mammals retain residual levels of these two enzymes and therefore retain some ability to use ketone bodies as fuel throughout life. Although ketone bodies can provide a significant level of brain ATP production, they cannot be used as the primary substrate. This is clearly shown by the inability of ketone bodies to restore brain function after the onset of hypoglycemic coma.

Since the normal brain requires a continuous supply of both glucose and oxygen, regardless of other circumstances, interruption of the supply of either substrate causes pathology. **Anoxia** begins to produce symptoms in ten to fifteen seconds, since there is no significant reserve of oxygen in the CNS. Given the high and continuous need for oxygen, even a brief interruption in the supply results in a loss of consciousness. The loss of consciousness is shortly followed by neuronal loss and consequent brain damage. Hypoxia and **ischemia** produce similar results, but with these conditions it takes longer for the damage to appear. Oxygen deficiency would be more serious and more rapid in onset than it is if it were not for a kind of a metabolic defense mechanism that amino acid metabolism provides. This defense mechanism was discussed in Chapter 4.

The response to a deficiency of glucose is similar, but less dramatic. A continuous supply of glucose is essential, even when ketone bodies are being consumed. If blood glucose is reduced from its normal level of about 4.5 mM to about 1 mM (about 18 mg per deciliter, or mg %), symptoms of hypoglycemia usually appear. Unlike the situation with oxygen, the brain does have a reserve, or buffer, of sources of ATP. Creatine phosphate is found in the brain, but it is not a major energy reserve. It has a high turnover rate, probably functioning as the primary source of energy instead of ATP for reactions that occur at a distance from mitochondria. Brain tissue contains significant (although not large) amounts of glycogen. Glycogen, which is composed of glucose, has a high turnover rate in the brain. It provides an effective energy reserve and can be used as an adequate source of glucose for several minutes. Despite the high fat content of the CNS, there is very little reserve of fat for energy purposes. The brain does not normally consume significant amounts of fat for energy.

By far the largest endogenous source of energy substrates is the pool of free amino acids. The brain is unique in that it contains a large amount of free amino acids (i.e., not bound in proteins). These are available for metabolism when glucose is in short supply. At such times, the amino acids are catabolized in the citric acid cycle and can supply a large amount of ATP.

All together, these endogenous reserves of energy will support the brain's needs for about half an hour. That is, if severe hypoglycemia has occurred, major symptoms may develop in less than an hour—a significantly longer time than it takes to develop symptoms of a shortage of oxygen.

GLUCOSE TRANSPORT

Considering the importance of the continuous glucose supply to the brain, the mechanism of glucose transport across the blood–brain barrier is important. Five different transporters for hexoses (six-carbon sugars), such as glucose, have been cloned and sequenced, four of which are specific for glucose. Two of these, GLUT1 and GLUT3, have been found in the CNS.

GLUT3 is not affected by insulin and apparently responds only to the relative concentrations of glucose on both sides of the membrane in which it resides. It is prominent in brain tissue, where it is likely concentrated in the membranes of neural cells. In this location, GLUT3 functions to equalize the concentration of glucose between the intra- and extracellular spaces. It facilitates transport to achieve this equilibrium.

It is traditional to regard all glucose transport into the brain as insulin-independent and therefore to assume that GLUT3 is the only glucose transporter active in the brain. GLUT4, the best-known insulin-regulated glucose transporter, has not been found in the brain. The GLUT1 transporter, however, is prominent in red cells, fetal tissue, and brain microvessels. Its presence in the blood supply to the brain suggests that it is a component of the blood–brain barrier. GLUT1 is regulated by insulin, although insulin's effect on GLUT1 is not as great as its effect on GLUT4.

It is not surprising that multiple glucose transporters exist within the CNS, as it is a highly complex tissue that uses more glucose proportionately than other tissues. Scientists have known for over twenty years (both from laboratory experiments in rodents and from human measurements) that insulin assists brain glucose uptake. There is also clinical evidence for insulin's usefulness in restoring normal brain metabolism in certain circumstances. For example, in the senile atherosclerotic patients with an RQ of 0.85 described above, digestion of their own brain substance was the likely explanation of the low RQ. In these patients, the addition of intravenous glucose alone did not restore brain RQ to normal, but giving both insulin and glucose restored the RQ to 0.99. This is an indication that, at least in some circumstances, insulin can be part of a beneficial therapeutic regimen for optimization of brain metabolism.

ACID REMOVAL

As mentioned earlier, blood flow in and out of the brain is critical, not only for supplying nutrients to the tissue but also for removing the large amount of CO_2 generated by the brain's metabolic processes. An interruption of blood flow, in even a small portion of the brain, results in energy starvation and an increased risk for the development of acidosis, both of which produce pathology.

When glucose first enters brain cells, it is metabolized in the cytoplasm by the enzymes of glycolysis. The main cytoplasmic product of glycolysis is pyruvic acid (pyruvate at normal pH). In normal circumstances, the pyruvate is oxidized in mitochondria to CO_2 and water. If mitochondrial metabolism is inhibited or overwhelmed, pyruvate and NADH build up in the cytoplasm. Pyruvate and NADH then form lactate, by the activity of lactate dehydrogenase. Lactate is often thought of as causing acidosis, and it does so under certain circumstances. Recent evidence, however, indicates that lactate and hydrogen ion concentrations (pH) do not always correlate with each other. A buildup of lactate does, however, seem to correlate with neuronal damage and loss of brain tissue, even when it does not correlate with low pH. Elevated lactate concentration is harmful, but is not always the source of brain acidosis.

Acidosis can also result when CO_2 is not adequately removed from the brain. The bicarbonate–carbon dioxide buffering system is the central physiological buffering system. Nearly all the CO_2 produced arises within the mitochondria, produced by reactions in the citric acid cycle. Therefore, in any condition in which the citric acid cycle continues to function beyond the capacity of the blood supply to remove its products, a CO_2-based acidosis can develop. Interruption of mitochondrial function (e.g., under conditions of O_2 deprivation) leads to a buildup of glycolytic products and intermediates, since the mitochondrion is necessary for their removal by metabolism. Therefore, in pathological circumstances, either too much or too little mitochondrial function can cause tissue damage. This issue is discussed further in Chapter 15.

THE REGULATION OF CEREBRAL BLOOD FLOW

Given the importance of the supply of energy substrate and of removal of metabolic waste products, the maintenance of adequate cerebral blood flow (CBF) is of vital importance for normal brain function. It has been known for some time that the primary mechanism for regulation of CBF is control of blood-vessel diameter: vasodilation increases blood flow, and vasoconstriction decreases it.

Attempts to understand the regulation of cerebral blood-vessel diameter have focused on metabolic control, because it is also known that neuronal activity and CBF are very tightly coupled. Energy metabolism, and CBF as well, increases with increased neuronal activity.

Lowering pH increases cerebral blood-vessel diameter, thus increasing blood flow. Increasing pCO_2 increases CBF (and also lowers pH). On the other hand, increasing pO_2 causes vasoconstriction, decreasing blood flow. These observations fit well with the view that brain metabolism regulates blood supply; high concentrations of oxygen (substrate) decrease CBF, and high concentrations of acids (products of metabolism) increase it. There are some difficulties with this view, however. The pH and blood gas changes that are required to modify CBF in vivo are relatively large, and it is not entirely clear that such fluctuations occur in vivo. These mechanisms may play a role in vivo only in extreme situations. Other CBF regulatory factors may be at work in vivo. Such modulators of neuronal activity as adenosine or nitric oxide (NO) may also be important. It is also possible that there are specific neurons, with processes ending on blood-vessel walls, that could directly regulate vessel diameter, and hence CBF, by releasing neuromodulators or transmitters. All of these possibilities, and others, are current topics of research.

Adenosine, which is possibly produced within all synapses in direct proportion to their activity (Chapter 3), can activate adenylyl cyclase and is probably a vasodilator. It is a product of the enzymatic degradation of ATP in the synaptic cleft. Both ATP and ADP have been shown to be generalized vasodilators, as well. ATP may be found within all synaptic vesicles, in which case it would be released along with the transmitter. Therefore, ATP may be released into extracellular fluid in proportion to total neurotransmitter release. Once outside the cell, it is metabolized to ADP and on to adenosine. It may be an important participant in the regulation of local CBF.

More recently, attention has focused on nitric oxide (NO), which may play a more important role in some parts of the CNS. NO is probably not produced at all synapses, since the enzyme that synthesizes it is not evenly distributed throughout the brain. Cells in the cerebellum, cerebral cortex, and other parts of the brain do contain NO synthetase. This enzyme is regulated by Ca^{++} concentration in combination with calmodulin. NO may be made within any cell that experiences a calcium influx in response to transmitter action. This means that any cell can produce NO if it contains NO synthetase and either NMDA receptors or the IP3 second-messenger system. In these cells, NO is produced in direct proportion to excitatory activity, is freely diffusible, and crosses cell membranes with ease. NO activates the soluble form of guanylyl cyclase, first binding to its associated heme group and then stimulating cyclic GMP synthesis from GTP. Interestingly, the NO produced in a particular cell will likely not activate cGMP synthesis in the same cell. NO production is stimulated by high Ca^{++} concentration, but Ca^{++} also inhibits guanylyl cyclase. NO production in one cell thus activates guanylyl cyclase in nearby cells, increasing the concentration of cyclic GMP in those cells that contain the soluble form of guanylyl cyclase and do not contain a high concentration of Ca^{++}. The cGMP produced by this reaction is a strong vasodilator. This mechanism could be a significant contributor to the regulation of CBF, at least in the areas of excitatory synapses. In this reaction NO is behaving as a hormone or transmitter, in that it affects cells other than those in which it is made (see Figure 14-1).

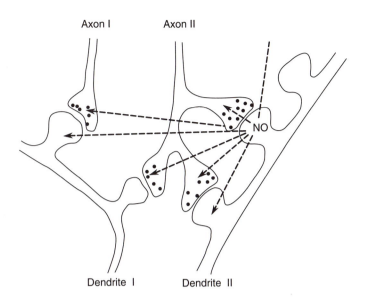

Figure 14-1 *Nitric oxide,
after being produced in
a single cell, is free to
diffuse to many nearby
synaptic terminals. It
may function in this way
to integrate the firing of
groups of terminals or
neurons.*

GLOBAL BRAIN METABOLISM

Interest in the mechanisms of integration of brain metabolism, synaptic function, and regional blood flow has increased since the discovery of the effect sometimes called the "cerebral steal" phenomenon. This phenomenon appears to be a "zero-sum" process for brain metabolism, whereby portions of the brain can change their metabolic rates, but the brain's total metabolic rate remains relatively unchanged. This phenomenon was first discovered by the use of radioactively labeled derivatives of glucose, which were taken up by brain regions in direct proportion to glucose uptake. The uptake can be measured in humans in vivo by a technique called Positron Emission Tomography (PET). Using PET, researchers observed that whenever one brain region became metabolically more active, another region of more or less comparable size decreased its rate of glucose uptake. For example, when a subject opens his or her eyes, the visual cortex increases its rate of glucose utilization while parts of the parietal and frontal regions decrease their glucose uptake. This zero-sum phenomenon has implications beyond those of the tight coupling of neuronal metabolism and local blood flow.

The zero sum for whole brain metabolism persists when neither the total amount of glucose nor oxygen availability is a limiting factor. In fact, in normal circumstances, only about 10 percent of available glucose is extracted from cerebral blood. Therefore, there must be some other limiting factor determining the whole brain metabolic rate. This mechanism, whatever it is, does not allow an increase in global brain energy metabolism when a single region is activated. This phenomenon and its mechanism are, at present, unknown but are of considerable interest.

METABOLISM AND COGNITION

Although its specific neuroanatomy and neurophysiology remain unknown, consciousness is generally believed to be a manifestation of global brain function.

Global brain metabolism and cognition, or level of consciousness of the organism, are coupled tightly together. This coupling may be the result of mechanisms separate from those that link local neuronal activity and blood flow. This coupling represents the sum of whole brain metabolism, including all the regional changes that might be taking place at any time. It may therefore be related to the zero-sum phenomenon.

At the cellular level, there is also a correlation between neuronal metabolism and function. As mentioned earlier, when neurons are resting, their metabolic rate is only about 60 percent of what it is when they are generating action potentials. It has also been mentioned that some depressant drugs (e.g., ethanol) inhibit the active metabolism component much more than they inhibit resting metabolism. It is possible that there is a relationship between the different kinds of metabolism at the cellular level and different levels of metabolism at the whole brain level.

A small (about 10 percent) depression of global brain metabolism produces clinically evident "confusion." A greater metabolic depression, approximately 25 to 40 percent, produces coma. (It is important to emphasize that coma can also be produced by functional deficits in specific regions of the brain, especially in the brainstem. The above-mentioned figures apply only to coma of a global origin.) This approximate relationship, between global brain metabolism and consciousness, is maintained whether the inhibition derives from general anesthesia, self-administered drugs, tumors, or trauma. Thus, there apparently is a narrow range within which brain metabolism can be modified without affecting mentation, but a large amount of "basic," or "resting," metabolism that is not directly related to consciousness.

Increases in whole brain metabolism can also occur, but only under very pathological conditions. For example, during seizures, especially during status epilepticus, there is a severalfold increase in brain metabolism. This increase may result in neural injury if it is prolonged, as the excessive metabolism of the cell can cause neuronal death and loss of brain substance.

In the absence of pathology, the maximum measured whole brain metabolic rate occurs during rapid eye movement (REM) sleep, and the minimum whole brain metabolic rate occurs during slow wave sleep (SWS). The difference between these two states and waking metabolism is only about 15 to 20 percent, with the waking period being intermediate. Therefore, the normal fluctuation in overall metabolic rate is quite small. The basal metabolic level of isolated neurons is sufficient to maintain the cells' survival for extended periods of time. A person in a coma, with decreased brain metabolism, may, in theory, have lost only the activated component of neuronal metabolism. Brain cells could survive under such circumstances indefinitely. Therefore, cerebral death cannot accurately be determined by physiological criteria (i.e., electroencephalography, or EEG) alone. The EEG measures only brain electrical activity. If the brain is electrically silent while the cells maintain metabolic activity (i.e., stay alive), other criteria must be used to determine death. A biochemical determination of cell viability would be highly desirable under these circumstances. Theoretically, such a biochemical assessment could be made by using the energy charge (EC):

$$EC = \frac{[ATP] + \frac{1}{2}[ADP]}{[ATP] + [ADP] + [AMP]}$$

This equation involves all three major adenine-containing nucleotides and has a theoretical range from 0 (when AMP is the only adenine ribonucleotide) to 1.0

(when ATP is the only adenine ribonucleotide). This ratio has been shown to be the major regulatory factor controlling all catabolism. The higher the EC, the more catabolism is inhibited and synthesis is stimulated. When the EC is low, synthesis is inhibited and catabolism is stimulated. The EC in normal brain tissue is about 0.95. It has been shown, in simple preparations, that a markedly diminished EC is a prelude to cell and tissue death. It is at least theoretically possible that EC determinations in the brain could be predictive of cell and tissue destruction and, therefore, of cerebral death. It is now possible to estimate the EC by modern, noninvasive techniques, such as (nuclear) magnetic resonance spectroscopy.

Because of the above considerations, when only physiological criteria such as the EEG are used to determine cerebral death, it is important not to apply them in cases of drug-induced comas. Since alcohol and barbiturates selectively inhibit the higher, activated level of metabolism, these drugs are capable of producing an isoelectric coma (i.e., a coma with no observable electrical activity) without actually killing the cells. Such cells can be thought of as "idling"—they are metabolically active but electrically silent. In fact, in one case a patient endured an isoelectric coma for more than forty hours and then recovered apparently normal function. Loss of activity does not mean loss of cells.

EXPERIMENTAL TECHNIQUES FOR MEASURING LOCAL BRAIN METABOLIC RATES

One of the most important techniques for measuring local brain metabolism, as opposed to global brain metabolism, uses 2-deoxyglucose (2-DG) (see Figure 14-2). The use of this molecule is based on its ability, because of its

Figure 14-2 The First Two Steps of Glycolysis

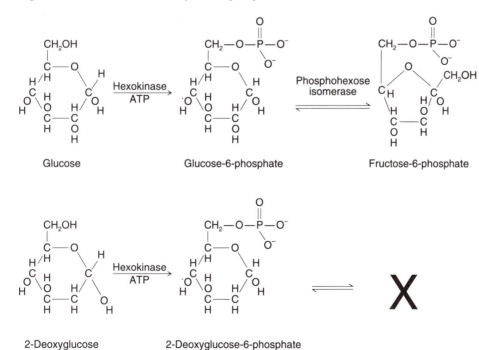

Glucose   Glucose-6-phosphate   Fructose-6-phosphate

2-Deoxyglucose   2-Deoxyglucose-6-phosphate

structural similarity to glucose, to be taken up by brain cells in direct proportion to their uptake of glucose. 2-DG uses many of the same membrane transporters as glucose. It also serves as a substrate for hexokinase, the first enzyme of intracellular glucose metabolism, which phosphorylates it. Once phosphorylated, it remains in the cellular compartment where the phosphorylation occurred, in this case, the cytosol. Phosphorylated molecules are not able to cross membranes without a specific transporter.

The second step in glycolysis is conversion of glucose-6-phosphate to fructose-6-phosphate, requiring the shift of a double bond from carbon 1 to carbon 2 (Figure 14-2). In the case of 2-deoxyglucose, the second carbon has no oxygen, so no shift is possible. This means that the phosphorylated 2-deoxyglucose can be metabolized no further and is trapped in this form. It cannot be metabolized, and it cannot leave the compartment. Since the amount of 2-deoxyglucose that entered the cell was directly proportional to the amount of glucose entering at the same time, the concentration of 2-deoxyglucose in the cell is directly proportional to the total glucose metabolism of that cell. If the 2-deoxyglucose is radioactively labeled, its presence in cells can be determined in vivo by PET. Regional cerebral metabolic rate can thus be measured in vivo without harming the individual. In this way, local glucose metabolic rates can be quantified. Data of this kind document the existence of the zero-sum phenomenon of brain metabolism, discussed above.

SELF-STUDY QUESTIONS

Facts:

1. Define RQ, gluconeogenesis, ketone body, and hypoglycemia.

2. Name the obligatory and supplementary energy substrates for CNS metabolism.

3. Name and describe the energy reserve molecules within the brain.

4. Describe the time course of brain damage following interruption of the supply of each obligatory substrate.

5. Describe the possible biochemical mechanisms for control of CBF, both in the brain as a whole and in specific foci.

Concepts:

1. Discuss the relationship between consciousness and metabolic rate.

2. Discuss the metabolic parameters that might be used to distinguish between coma and brain death.

3. Discuss the relationship between insulin's effects and CNS metabolism.

4. Discuss the implications of RQ across the brain.

5. Discuss the mechanism of the 2-deoxyglucose technique of metabolism assessment.

BIBLIOGRAPHY

Atkinson, D. 1977. *Cellular Energy Metabolism and Its Regulation*. New York: Academic Press.

Benzel, E.C., and Wild, G.C. 1991. Biochemical mechanisms of posttraumatic neural injury. *Perspect. Neurol. Surg*. 2: 95–126.

Clarke, D.D., Lajtha, A.L., and Maker, H.S. 1989. Intermediary metabolism. In *Basic Neurochemistry*, edited by G. Siegel, B.W. Agranoff, R.W. Albers, and P. Molinoff. New York: Raven Press.

Ingvar, D.H., and Lassen, N.A., eds. 1975. *Brain Work: The Coupling of Function, Metabolism and Blood Flow in the Brain*. Copenhagen: Munsk-gaard.

Sokoloff, L. 1989. Circulation and energy metabolism of the brain. In *Basic Neurochemistry*, edited by G. Siegel, B.W. Agranoff, R.W. Albers, and P. Molinoff. New York: Raven Press.

Medical Neurochemistry

CHAPTER 15

Acid–Base Balance and CNS Injury

Acid–base balance in the CNS is maintained by many of the fundamental mechanisms used in other tissues, but the process is unique in the CNS because of the blood–brain barrier and the tissue's high metabolic rate. Maintaining pH becomes a more significant problem after injury, as the CNS may be at risk for a life-threatening acidosis. Therefore, metabolism, the major pH buffering systems of the brain, and the regulatory mechanisms for each of these are of major clinical importance.

NORMAL CNS METABOLISM

Energy metabolism in brain tissue is fundamentally similar to that in other tissues, with the exceptions noted in Chapter 14. Since glucose metabolism accounts for nearly all ATP production in the brain, it also accounts for nearly all acid production. Glycolysis takes place in cytoplasm, being regulated by the energy charge (Chapter 14) and producing ATP, pyruvate, and NADH. Normally, most of the pyruvate is transported into nearby mitochondria, where it is oxidized to CO_2 and H_2O, with the concomitant production of large amounts of reduced nucleotide cofactors. These reduced cofactors are then reoxidized by the electron transport system, leading to the production of the bulk of the ATP (and H_2O) that glucose provides to the tissue (Figure 15-1).

A single glucose molecule yields in the range of thirty-six molecules of ATP and six molecules of carbon dioxide when completely catabolized. All of the CO_2 and nearly all of the ATP are made in the mitochondria. A small amount of ATP (about 5 percent of the total) is produced in the cytoplasm. Therefore, glucose metabolism in the brain requires that both cellular compartments, mitochondria and cytoplasm, work in accord.

Other energy substrates, such as ketone bodies, amino acids, and fatty acids, can be oxidized by the brain in some circumstances. All of these substrates are metabolized nearly completely within mitochondria, without significant cytoplasmic catabolism. These substrates are also oxidized completely to CO_2 and H_2O.

This metabolic compartmentation is significant for the production of acid and its possible damage to brain cells. The bulk of CNS acid is mitochondrial and

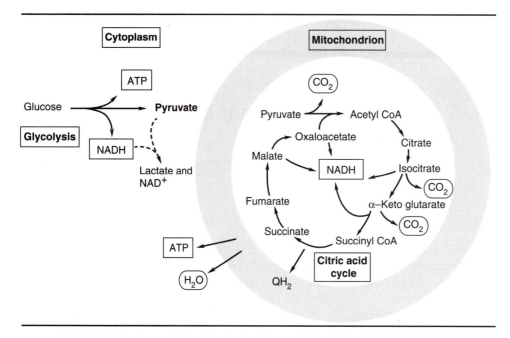

Figure 15-1 The Compartmentation of Catabolism in Neurons

is in the form of CO_2, the acid part of the bicarbonate–carbon dioxide buffer system. The equation for this relationship is:

$$pH = pK + \log \frac{[HCO_3^-]}{\alpha \times pCO_2}$$

This is the Henderson–Hasselbalch equation, in its most appropriate form for CO_2 buffers in biological systems. The pCO_2 stands for the partial pressure of CO_2 (gas) dissolved in the system, as this is more significant than the concentration of carbonic acid (H_2CO_3). The pK (6.1) used is that for the system from CO_2 to HCO_3^-. The α (alpha) is a constant for converting the gas pressure to mM ($\alpha = 0.031$). As this equation shows, as pCO_2 rises, pH drops. CO_2, being produced in all mitochondria in large quantities, must be quickly removed from the CNS or it will create an acidotic state.

In addition, if mitochondria are damaged or metabolically overwhelmed, glucose metabolism in cytoplasm will cause a buildup of pyruvate. The pyruvate combines with NADH (also produced in cytoplasm by glycolysis) to form lactate. Lactate may have a toxicity beyond its contribution to a lower pH. There is evidence that cellular lactate concentration correlates with neuronal death, even in circumstances when the lactate concentration does not correlate with pH.

Metabolic Regulation

All of this catabolism, involving multiple enzymes and cellular compartments, is normally tightly controlled by several different types and stages of regulatory processes. There are multiple levels of regulation, from short-term allosteric mechanisms, through covalent modification, to long-term changes in the amount of enzymes produced by regulation of the genes that express them. Most regulations of catabolism, at all levels, are in the homeostatic, negative feedback (NFB) direction. That is, when ATP production is too high, catabolism is inhibited, and ATP concentration then falls. When ATP production rises, synthesis increases, and catabolism is inhibited. Synthesis uses ATP, and as its concentration falls, catabolism is stimulated again.

There are, however, several ways in which NFB mechanisms can be overridden. Many hormones produce changes in enzymes that will override allosteric NFB inhibition. The changes often take the form of covalent modifications (e.g., phosphorylation) of the allosteric enzymes. There are also other allosteric mechanisms that can override NFB, which have been most thoroughly studied in the liver. One mechanism for this type of override, called positive feed forward (PFF), is the system used by the liver to make fat from carbohydrate. This process most commonly takes place as the result of an excess consumption of carbohydrate. If NFB were to work perfectly, it would not be possible to store energy beyond one's immediate needs.

PFF works via the allosteric enzymes that control glycolysis. Phosphofructokinase (PFK) is the primary NFB regulator of glycolysis, and pyruvate kinase (PK) is the site of the primary regulation of PFF. PK is the third, and last, allosteric enzyme in glycolysis.

Substrate Availability and Delivery

The transport of glucose across the blood–brain barrier was discussed in Chapter 14. The GLUT3 transporter is not affected by insulin and is found in large quantity in the brain. It may be the transporter via which glucose moves from extracellular fluid (ECF) into cells. The GLUT1 transporter, on the other hand, is affected by insulin. It has also been found in the brain and constitutes part of the blood–brain barrier. Therefore, insulin likely has an effect on glucose's entry into the brain from blood, but not on its entry into neurons from ECF. This point has been widely misunderstood, but this compartmentation now seems clear.

Cerebral Blood Flow and Cellular Metabolism

Regional cerebral blood flow (rCBF) and regional cellular metabolism are tightly coupled, sufficiently so that changes in neuronal metabolism are now routinely used to indicate changes in rCBF (Chapter 14). It is possible for the two to become uncoupled, however. The specific mechanisms by which the coupling is determined and maintained are not well known. Therefore, the mechanisms for the uncoupling of CBF and cellular metabolism are also unknown. The major hypotheses for the coupling include pH, pO_2, pCO_2, adenosine, and NO as coupling agents (Chapter 14). Other mechanisms are also possible.

Despite the fact that glycolysis and the citric acid cycle occur in separate compartments of the cell, and that both normally operate at higher levels in the brain than in any other tissue, there has been little investigation of their coupling in the CNS. In many parts of the neuron, there must be a significant uncoupling of these two pathways, since mitochondria are not as evenly distributed throughout the cell as is cytoplasm. Both pathways are controlled by complex regulatory systems, which are somewhat separate from each other. It is possible, then, that either pathway could be inhibited more than the other or stimulated more than the other under different circumstances. In such unbalanced circumstances, the potential exists for metabolically induced damage, either by overproduction of waste products (e.g., lactate and CO_2) or by underproduction of energy.

Acid–Base Balance in the CNS

As discussed above, the fundamental mechanisms of acid–base balance in the CNS are similar to those in other tissues, with two major exceptions. One exception is the presence of the blood–brain barrier. This barrier is primarily against ions, large molecules, and cells and prevents or slows their movement from blood to brain, or vice versa. The CO_2 buffering system is the main such system in the body. The numerator of the Henderson–Hasselbalch equation is an ion, bicarbonate, which does not cross the blood–brain barrier easily. The denominator, on the other hand, is CO_2, a relatively non-polar molecule that is a gas at room temperature. CO_2 crosses membranes readily.

One consequence of these facts is that treatment of acidosis in blood can worsen the acidosis in the CNS. If an acidosis is treated by infusing bicarbonate, the bicarbonate will raise the numerator of the equation, and hence raise the pH of the bloodstream. The bicarbonate is prevented from crossing the blood–brain barrier, however, so it cannot change the acid–base ratio in the CNS. Carbonic anhydrase converts the bicarbonate anion to H_2CO_3 and, therefore, to CO_2. H_2CO_3 is an unstable molecule, breaking down quickly in solution to water and carbon dioxide. Some elevation of CO_2 will therefore also occur in blood due to the diffusion of the CO_2 back across the blood–brain barrier.

$$HCO_3^- + H^+ \rightleftharpoons [H_2CO_3] \rightleftharpoons H_2O + CO_2$$

The CO_2 is able to cross the blood–brain barrier, entering the CNS and increasing the denominator of the fraction. Therefore, in the acidotic patient treated with bicarbonate, pH in the CNS may be lowered.

CNS anatomy is such that, whereas the blood supply to the CNS is adequate for its metabolic needs, isolated areas of the CNS are separated by some distance from the nearest blood vessels. One consequence of this arrangement is the dependence of these areas on diffusion of small molecules. Glucose must diffuse from the nearest blood vessel to each cell and pyruvate must diffuse to each cell's mitochondria. Oxygen must diffuse from the blood vessel to mitochondria. Conversely, CO_2 and H_2O, the products of metabolism, must diffuse back to the blood vessel. A buildup of either metabolic waste product in a particular region or cell can be the cause of pathology.

INJURY TO THE CNS

Primary Injury

A primary CNS injury arises from one (or a combination) of three fundamental causes: (1) disruption of cellular integrity, (2) distortion of the cell, and/or (3) metabolic derangement(s). Any of these may result in the death or temporary or permanent dysfunction of the cell. Therapeutic intervention is most frequently required for cell distortion and metabolic aberrations, as these are the most common causes of neurological injury. Any significant disruption usually results in cell death. Extreme distortion of the cell may also result in ischemia and abnormalities in nutrient and metabolite diffusion.

Secondary Injury

Secondary injury may be defined as "an injury to a neuron and its supporting cells that is delayed, thus following a primary neurologic insult by a finite period of time. This injury results in a cell dropout (death) that is greater than that observed with the primary injury alone." Secondary injury is perhaps more of a metabolic phenomenon than primary injury, whereas primary injury may be only mechanical disruption or distortion of the cell. Secondary injury, since it is complex and takes place over a longer period of time than primary injury, may be more susceptible to therapeutic interventions.

The demarcation between the primary and the secondary injury is not always clear. For example, if cell distortion results in a cell's death at some time following the primary injury, the cell's death may be related to either the primary *or* the secondary injury. Tissue damage following CNS injury, including stroke, traumatic brain injury (TBI), and spinal cord injury (SCI), reflects both primary and secondary injuries.

Reperfusion injury is a different pathological process that is similar in some ways to secondary injury. Reperfusion injury is the name given to the cell death that occurs not at the time of blockage of blood flow (such as in a stroke), but in a burst during the period when blood flow is first reintroduced to the ischemic zone. It is now clear that many tissues may suffer as much, or even more, damage during the initial reperfusion process than during the period of ischemia.

Ongoing Primary Injury

When cells suffer ongoing injury (such as ischemia), it can sometimes be difficult to differentiate between ongoing primary and secondary injury. Many degenerative neurologic diseases, such as atherosclerosis, senile dementia, and others, fit into this category. Ongoing primary injury implies the possibility of ongoing secondary injury. If, for example, ongoing ischemia in the region surrounding a stroke persists for several days, the secondary injury may last for several days. Similarly, if the ongoing primary injury is indefinite, such as with Alzheimer's disease, the secondary injury may last indefinitely. The timing and duration of therapy need to be adjusted appropriately.

Numerous fundamental processes must be more clearly understood before primary, ongoing primary, and secondary injury phenomena are sorted out and effectively treated.

BIOCHEMICAL MECHANISMS OF THE SECONDARY INJURY RESPONSE

Free Radical Production

The theory that the secondary injury results from **free radicals** is popular at present. The term "free radical" is given to any chemical species that contains at least one unpaired electron and thus tends to be reactive. Free radicals are uncommon in biological systems because most of the atoms in biological molecules have shared or lost their unpaired electrons before gaining biological usefulness. There are important exceptions to this generalization, however. Oxygen itself is a di-radical; the most common form of molecular, atmospheric oxygen contains two unpaired electrons. Therefore, oxygen, the basis of all animal life, is highly spontaneously reactive and is a biological toxin.

Many other oxygen-containing molecules are also free radicals. The hydroxyl radical ($\cdot$OH) is the most reactive such intermediate and is therefore the most toxic. (Note that the hydroxyl radical is distinct from the hydroxide ion, OH^-, which is not a radical.) Free radical damage to cells results from the radicals' high reactivity and the fact that, in most cases, this reaction produces one or more free radicals. This creates a chain reaction, resulting in continuous production of free radicals. The chain proceeds until it is broken.

Unsaturated fatty acids, found in high concentration in mammalian cell membranes, are especially vulnerable to free radicals. Such a fatty acid reacts with a radical, producing a fatty acid derivative that cannot be further metabolized. The reaction produces other toxic molecules, such as malondialdehyde. Malondialdehyde is not a free radical; it is toxic because it is also highly reactive with biological molecules. Aldehydes cross-link protein molecules, thus "fixing" them. (Formaldehyde is used for embalming because it exhibits this property.) Molecules such as malondialdehyde, having two aldehyde groups on each molecule, are especially potent in this kind of cell fixation.

Some biological molecules protect against free radical injury. They react with the unpaired electron and become stable free radicals themselves. This stability stops the chain reaction, ending the toxic effects. Vitamin E (alpha tocopherol) is an example of such a protective molecule. As oxygen consumption rises, the flux of oxygen through the tissue increases. The greater the amount of oxygen in the tissue, the greater the amount of **spontaneous** oxygen radical formation. Similarly, if the content of unsaturated fatty acids in the tissue rises, the possibility of free radical chain reactions increases. In either situation, the spontaneous production of free radicals is augmented by increasing the concentration of reactants. In both situations, the dietary requirement for vitamin E increases, in order to offset the harmful effects of the free radicals.

Other biological molecules are associated with free radical production. Uric acid (urate at normal pH) is the metabolic end product of the turnover of all purine residues in the body, whether from the diet or from endogenous synthesis. Large amounts of urate are produced in the CNS, where the turnover of purines is extraordinarily high. The enzyme that catalyzes urate formation is xanthine oxidase (XO), which also catalyzes other important biological reactions. The XO reaction uses oxygen as one substrate, in addition to purine. XO produces hydrogen peroxide (H_2O_2) in addition to urate. Hydrogen peroxide is one of the naturally occurring toxic metabolites of oxygen. The body contains several enzymes that can degrade it to less toxic substances. Catalase generates water and oxygen from H_2O_2; glutathione peroxidase forms water and oxidized glutathione. Both enzymes detoxify hydrogen peroxide by destroying it. But, as with oxygen, when hydrogen peroxide is increased over time, the likelihood of spontaneous reactions also increases. One hydrogen peroxide molecule can spontaneously form *two* hydroxyls ($\cdot$OH), the most toxic of all oxygen metabolites. Therefore, an increase in urate production results in an obligatory increase in hydrogen peroxide, as well as an increased likelihood of hydroxyl formation.

Glutathione metabolism is affected by the toxic intermediates of oxygen, as mentioned above. Reduced glutathione is needed by all cells to maintain the reduced environment of the cytoplasm. Either hydrogen peroxide or other organic peroxides that form as by-products of oxygen's presence in tissue can be catabolized to harmless products by glutathione peroxidase. The reaction also converts reduced glutathione to oxidized glutathione. Therefore, increasing the amount of hydrogen peroxide decreases the concentration of glutathione.

Free radicals and toxic oxygen metabolites have been implicated in many kinds of CNS damage. They are thought to play a role in many chronic conditions, such as Parkinson's disease and normal aging, as well as in many situations involving acute injury. For example, the release of both urate and vitamin E from the spinal cord is increased following autoimmune damage to the CNS. The release of reduced glutathione, on the other hand, is decreased. These are the changes that would be expected if free radicals had arisen in the tissue during the autoimmune attack. (Many chronic diseases, such as multiple sclerosis, are thought to be autoimmune in origin.) Similar changes may occur in ischemia.

Nitric Oxide and the Superoxide Anion

Recent discoveries have focused attention on nitric oxide (NO) as a possible mechanism for the secondary injury response (Chapters 3 and 14). NO is a simple molecule. It contains only two atoms and is a gas at room temperature. It is also a free radical, although not a highly reactive one. NO appears to be one of the most powerful regulators in biological systems, especially in blood vessels, brain, and kidney.

NO is made in the cytoplasm from the free amino acid arginine, by NO synthetase. The products of the reaction are the amino acid citrulline and NO. Citrulline can then be reconverted to arginine in many cells. NO synthesis is stimulated by Ca^{++} complexed to calmodulin. Once formed, NO is free to diffuse out of the cell and can stimulate guanylyl cyclase and other enzymes in other cells. NO has many properties of a hormone or a neurotransmitter; it is made in one cell and affects others (Chapter 14). NO has also been shown to have cellular protective effects in myocardial ischemia, during the reperfusion. Yet in other cells, such as leukocytes, NO may have a role in the killing of foreign cells. Although the picture is still somewhat confused, and many details of NO's role have yet to be established, NO is clearly an important modulator in biological systems, including the brain.

Scientists have speculated for some time that the superoxide anion ($\cdot O_2^-$), another free radical form of partially reduced oxygen, could be the mechanism for much of the secondary injury response and for reperfusion injury in several tissues. Although the hydroxyl radical ($\cdot OH$) is known to be the most reactive of oxygen's metabolites, superoxide has been aggressively studied for its role in delayed injury, especially in the brain and heart. It is believed to initiate free radical chain reactions in membrane lipids. There is recent evidence, however, that at least some of the toxicity of superoxide may be due to its interaction with NO rather than to its generalized free radical reactivity. This evidence is supported by two facts: (1) superoxide is not a highly reactive free radical, and (2) it is highly reactive with

NO, destroying NO in the process. If NO has a protective function in the brain, as it does in the heart, the destruction of NO by superoxide might explain some of superoxide's toxicity. The reaction of superoxide and nitric oxide also produces hydroxyl free radicals, which are certainly damaging.

Excitotoxins

A generalized release of glutamate and other excitatory amino acid transmitters has been shown to occur in response to many types of tissue damage. The excitatory amino acid transmitters, glutamate, aspartate, and their derivatives, are capable of exciting neurons to the point of self-destruction (Chapter 10). The mechanism of excitotoxic cell injury is related to Ca^{++} flux into the cell. Increased concentrations of intracellular Ca^{++} have manifold effects, resulting from calcium's role as an allosteric modifier of a wide variety of enzymes. Excess intracellular Ca^{++} is now thought to be one of the major effectors of cell death and may be the common cause of cell death in many different situations. As NMDA receptors are a major source of intracellular calcium, the use of NMDA antagonists may be therapeutic in some circumstances. In fact, NMDA antagonists have been clinically reported to improve neurological outcome after CNS injury.

IMPEDIMENTS TO BLOOD FLOW

CNS tissue distortion, decreased cerebral perfusion, and edema (which impedes **interstitial** diffusion) all restrict the delivery of energy substrates to the cell and the dissipation of the waste products away from the cell. Therapeutic interventions seek to optimize oxygen and glucose delivery and removal of waste products and toxins, thus minimizing the primary as well as the secondary injury.

GLUCOSE METABOLISM AND NEURAL INJURY

Too much or too little available glucose may be harmful to neural tissue. Diminished intracellular glucose levels (i.e., hypoglycemia) are known to cause cell injury or dysfunction. It has also been shown that elevated glucose, near the time of the injury, appears to increase the extent of neural damage (see below).

If at least some collateral flow is available, brain glucose concentration correlates with serum glucose level. During ischemia, the flux of glucose into the cell increases. This provides increased substrate for glycolysis and, thus, for the production of lactate. The importance of having some collateral blood flow during ischemia cannot be overemphasized. Collateral flow is essential for cell survival in the region of the **penumbra** (the area surrounding the focus of damage) after ischemia. Experimental animals who experience a total cessation of blood flow in the penumbra show no response to changes in blood glucose after the onset of the ischemia. This is expected, since glucose cannot reach the brain cells if there is no blood flow to them.

Serum glucose levels and CNS tissue glucose levels most likely correlate following neurotrauma, as they do after focal cerebral ischemia, if there is some collateral flow. Therefore, some parallels of metabolism and treatment can be expected. Glucose metabolism has been intensively studied in connection with stroke, both in animals and in humans. There is a direct correlation between the extent of the neurological injury and the serum glucose levels at the time of the injury. Furthermore, insulin treatment around the time of the injury, producing a lowered blood glucose, has been observed to decrease infarction size and neurological injury. These observations have been made under a variety of experimental conditions, both in experimental animals and in humans.

There are several possible mechanisms for these effects. Insulin, by increasing the transport of serum glucose into muscle and other tissues, might decrease the amount of glucose in brain tissue, and hence the accumulation of lactate. Other mechanisms are also possible. These include the possibility of a direct, beneficial effect of insulin on the CNS. Insulin does increase glucose transport across the blood–brain barrier, using the GLUT1 transporter. It is also possible that insulin has a beneficial effect on damaged tissue that is different from (i.e., greater than) its effect on the intact brain. Insulin also enhances anabolism by mechanisms other than glucose transport. It is possible that the beneficial effect is due to increased anabolism, independent of glucose. Therefore, a variety of insulin effects could be factors in its improvement of neurological outcome following CNS injury.

Insufficient Glucose and Neural Damage

When inadequate supplies of energy substrates are available to the CNS, it can, and does, utilize endogenous substrates. This process is obviously limited. These mechanisms help the brain resist damage resulting from short-term substrate deprivation. The brain contains a reserve of one or two minutes' worth of glycogen and fats. Amino acids provide an endogenous energy supply for about half an hour. When endogenous supplies are exhausted and inadequate amounts of glucose are being delivered by blood, cell injury may occur. Under these conditions, metabolism may actually begin to digest vital portions of the cells, leading to their deaths. Either too little glucose (hypoglycemia) or too high an energy demand (as in epilepsy) can cause cell death.

It is not clear which specific enzymes are overstimulated in these situations or which substrates they are digesting. If either glycolysis or the citric acid cycle were to be stimulated to the point of requiring more than the available glucose and endogenous substrates, membrane lipid hydrolysis could occur, either by lysosomes or by extralysosomal enzymes. Acidosis, which commonly occurs after injury, activates lysosomes. Ischemia, by a presumably independent mechanism, has been shown to activate extralysosomal enzymes. If membrane lipids are digested in either case, harm to the cell results. It has in fact been shown that phospholipase A2 (PLA2) is activated by ischemia, and specifically hydrolyzes phosphoinositides in neuronal membranes. This process degrades membrane lipids (and also produces prostaglandins and other eicosanoids).

Excess Glucose and Neural Damage

There are several possible mechanisms by which glucose could exacerbate CNS injury. They include lactate production, osmotic effects, positive feed forward (PFF)–induced acidosis, enhancement of cholinergic effects, and effects of other toxic by-products, such as nitrogen-containing molecules. The fact that acidosis commonly accompanies neural injury implies that the catabolism of glucose exceeds the rate of removal of acidic products. This imbalance could be due either to mitochondrial metabolism that is insufficient to handle the products of glycolysis or to inadequate fluid flow to remove carbon dioxide and other acids.

On the other hand, an increased catabolism of glucose can augment the anabolic repair processes, if it is coupled to ATP production (i.e., oxidative phosphorylation). A discrepancy between, or an uncoupling of, glucose metabolism and oxygen consumption could be a crucial factor in determining whether glucose metabolism is harmful or beneficial during injury.

Acid and Lactate Production

A commonly held theory regarding the mechanism of hyperglycemia-induced neural injury is that lactate production from cytoplasmic glycolysis causes acidosis and therefore cell damage. There is considerable evidence available to indicate that acidosis is important in CNS damage following stroke. It is not so clear, however, that lactate is the source of the acidosis. As mentioned above, pH may vary independently from lactate concentration in the CNS. Although excessive lactate production can certainly result in lowered pH, it may not be the predominant factor regarding CNS acidification in many circumstances. Lactate concentration and pH may be independent of each other, but lactate alone may be directly toxic in concentrations above about 17 mM. These levels have been shown to be associated with cell death.

Lactate buildup is often a manifestation of mitochondrial insufficiency. If the mitochondria are overwhelmed, have been damaged, or are metabolically dysfunctional for any reason (e.g., hypoxia or anoxia), pyruvate and lactate will build up because pyruvate cannot be oxidized. When pyruvate and lactate are produced in unusually large quantities (e.g., as a result of a PFF mechanism), their concentrations will build up only if mitochondrial capacity is not sufficient to handle the increase. In any case, mitochondrial dysfunction should be considered as a likely primary problem.

During normal CNS metabolism, mitochondria are the major source of CO_2 and, therefore, of biological acid. CO_2 is produced at a high rate because of the high CNS demand for ATP. After trauma or tissue damage, there is increased protein and membrane lipid degradation due to an increase in lysosomal activity and possibly the activity of other enzymes. The amino acid and fatty acid products of this degradation are all substrates for mitochondrial metabolism, resulting in increased CO_2 production.

Besides being the basis of the main acid–base buffering system in biology, CO_2 also has the ability to bind nonenzymatically to proteins. This binding changes the regulatory and functional properties of the proteins involved. Therefore, excess CO_2 production (at levels beyond the capacity of the vascular system) can cause considerable neural damage, both by acidification and by protein modification. Thus, mitochondrial production of CO_2 may contribute substantially to the overall metabolic acid production.

The Osmotic Effect

A high glucose concentration in the extracellular fluid at the time of CNS injury could produce an osmotic effect that is damaging to neural cells, drawing out water and leaving the cells dehydrated. In normal circumstances, the cytoplasm of cells is about 36–46 M in water, as opposed to 55.6 M for pure water. This may represent a minimal intracellular water concentration, with further dehydration being harmful. Osmotically dehydrated cells may not be able to respond appropriately to trauma and may be at greater risk of death as a result. This hypothesis is unlikely in the case of hyperglycemia following neurotrauma, because the osmotic increase of glucose is likely not great enough to produce a significant effect. Nevertheless, this is an area for further research.

Positive Feed Forward Mechanisms

In order for high intracellular glucose concentrations to have short-term toxic effects other than its effects on osmotic pressure, the glucose must be metabolized. Elevated serum glucose concentrations might not be expected to increase metabolism inside neural cells because of the numerous NFB regulatory mechanisms discussed above. Intracellular glucose concentrations are already known to be higher (about 1–1.5 mM) than those of all other intermediates of intermediary metabolism. This is ten to one hundred times higher than that of other metabolic intermediates (typically 10–100 μM). These data imply that glucose concentration is not rate-limiting under normal circumstances. Increasing the concentration of glucose in the extracellular fluid, and consequently inside neurons as well, might stimulate its own metabolism. This could exacerbate CNS injury by acidosis and by excessive lactate accumulation. Increased glucose in liver cells does lead to increased glucose metabolism; a similar phenomenon may exist in brain cells.

If increasing glucose concentration were to increase glucose catabolism, a PFF mechanism would have to exist. There is no direct evidence regarding the existence of PFF mechanisms in the CNS, but certain observations suggest that they do, indeed, exist. Memory formation is enhanced, both in laboratory animals and in humans, by increasing serum glucose. This indicates that increasing serum glucose levels produces functional changes in the brain. It also implies a PFF mechanism (or mechanisms) in the brain.

Inhibitors of glycolysis have been shown to prevent the worsening of outcomes caused by elevated glucose in the blood at the time of stroke. This also implies that excess serum glucose is being metabolized, again presumably by a PFF mechanism.

If a PFF mechanism exists in the brain only for glycolysis, then lactate and pyruvate will accumulate. If the citric acid cycle is also affected, CO_2 will accumulate. In either case the accumulated waste products will harm the cell.

GLUCOSE ASSISTANCE IN NEURAL REPAIR

Following the line of reasoning used above, we must assume that there are circumstances in which elevated glucose could be helpful to neurological outcome and, therefore, could increase cell survival. Two major hypotheses attempt to explain this beneficial effect: (1) enhanced cholinergic activity and (2) enhanced anabolic activity.

Enhanced Cholinergic Activity

It has been suggested that glucose enhancement of learning is related to augmented cholinergic activity. Acetylcholine stimulates some of the brain nuclei involved in learning and, therefore, could be a direct effector. Drugs that are cholinergic agonists produce effects similar to those of elevated glucose. It is, therefore, possible that one effect is working by means of the other. Another possibility is that elevated glucose concentrations cause an increase in acetylcholine synthesis and release. This hypothesis also requires a PFF mechanism. Acetylcholine is made from acetyl CoA and choline by the enzyme choline acetyl transferase (ChAT) (Chapter 5). The acetyl group comes from glucose, by way of glycolysis and the mitochondrion. This hypothesis predicts that increasing glucose concentration can increase acetyl CoA production and thereby increase acetylcholine synthesis. However, it has been known for years that the rate-limiting factor in acetylcholine synthesis is choline availability (Chapter 5). It is not clear how an increase in acetyl CoA could increase the amount of acetylcholine produced. This hypothesis requires more direct data before it can be considered probable.

Enhanced Anabolic Activity

It is also possible that elevated glucose levels increase ATP production and raise the energy charge of the cell. This, in turn, would increase anabolism. The data that increased serum glucose enhances learning imply that it increases de novo syntheses of RNA, protein, and a variety of synaptic lipids. All of these syntheses are known to be necessary for long-term memory consolidation. It is possible that increased brain glucose produces and maintains an enhanced energy charge sufficient to support long-term learning. A similar effect of increased glucose could be helpful during the reparative phase following neurotrauma. Reparative processes require increased synthesis of the same classes of macromolecules essential to learning. Enhanced glucose metabolism might stimulate this process.

Several of these hypotheses require a PFF mechanism in neural tissue. As mentioned, the facts that glucose enhances learning, that increased glucose at the time of stroke worsens acidosis and outcome, and that glycolytic inhibitors reverse the negative effect of increased blood glucose during stroke all imply that such a PFF mechanism exists in the brain. Such PFF mechanisms could be either harmful (if they increase acidosis) or helpful (if they increase the energy charge and enhance anabolism).

THE TIMING OF GLUCOSE'S EFFECTS

Because of the above considerations, it is not appropriate to assume that the presence of glucose following neural injury is necessarily bad. This is a common clinical assumption, based on the data demonstrating the harmful effects of high concentrations of glucose at the time of injury. In fact, the relationship between serum glucose and neural injury is complex. It includes all facets of glucose availability and utilization, many of which have been discussed above. There are almost certainly times when glucose is "bad," because it contributes to acidosis or the buildup of other toxins. Conversely, there are probably also times when glucose is "good," because it enhances anabolism. The accurate definition of these time periods would seem to be of considerable importance for the development of appropriate interventions, and therefore this is a topic for further research.

It is likely that increased glucose during the first hour or two following neural injury augments the injury, as is true after stroke. However, following this initial time period, it is possible that there is a time when increased glucose enhances anabolism, neural repair, and recovery. Augmenting glucose availability during this time period would lead to increased cell survival and improved functional outcome.

Therefore, increased glucose can be a part of either damage or therapy. Given what is now known about the response of neural tissue to trauma, it seems reasonable to postulate that both kinds of sequelae can and do occur.

SUMMARY AND RECOMMENDATIONS FOR FUTURE RESEARCH

The timing of glucose supplementation is critical following CNS injury. Acidosis and lactate production are damaging, and tissue anabolism is beneficial. It appears that the early administration of glucose following injury worsens acidosis and increases lactate production. This practice is therefore harmful. Conversely, the administration of glucose at a later time encourages anabolic cellular repair and is therefore beneficial. The precise time frames during which these events occur are not established at present.

More information is needed regarding the different phases of neural metabolism during and following the time of injury. Multiple questions, each one a subject for future research projects, may be asked. During which time period is glucose administration harmful, and conversely, when is it helpful? Does PFF occur in neurons? Does PFF drive neurons to self-destruction, and if so, how? What are the consequences of the uncoupling of CBF from neuronal firing and of the glycolytic pathway from mitochondrial metabolism? What are the consequences of interfering with, or increasing, the production of NO? If PFF mechanisms exist in brain metabolism, what advantage do they provide? What are the roles of the blood–brain barrier and of GLUT1 transport in the CNS? Finally, how are the accepted mechanisms of the secondary injury response (such as free radical production or excitotoxicity) related to cellular catabolic processes?

SELF-STUDY QUESTIONS

Facts:

1. Describe negative feedback and positive feed forward.

2. Name the metabolic sources of CNS acid.

3. What are the differences between GLUT1 and GLUT3?

Concepts:

1. Explain the mechanism by which treating a peripheral acidosis with bicarbonate can worsen acidosis in the CNS.

169
Self-Study Questions

2. What evolutionary advantage is provided to the CNS by having insulin-assisted glucose transport from blood into ECF, but not from ECF into neurons?

3. If it is true that hyperglycemia increases CNS anabolism, what implications does this have for diabetes?

BIBLIOGRAPHY

Atkinson, D. 1977. *Cellular Energy Metabolism and Its Regulation*. New York: Academic Press.

Benzel, E.C., and Wild, G.C. 1991. Biochemical mechanisms of posttraumatic neural injury. *Perspect. Neurol. Surg.* 2: 95–126.

Clarke, D.D., Lajtha, A.L., and Maker, H.S. 1989. Intermediary metabolism. In *Basic Neurochemistry,* edited by G. Siegel, B.W. Agranoff, R.W. Albers, and P. Molinoff. New York: Raven Press.

Ingvar, D.H., and Lassen, N.A., eds. 1975. *Brain Work: The Coupling of Function, Metabolism and Blood Flow in the Brain*. Copenhagen: Munskgaard.

Siesjo, B.K. 1988. Acidosis and ischemic brain damage. *Neurochemical Pathology* 9: 31–88.

Sokoloff, L. 1989. Circulation and energy metabolism of the brain. In *Basic Neurochemistry*, edited by G. Siegel, B.W. Agranoff, R.W. Albers, and P. Molinoff. New York: Raven Press.

CHAPTER 16

The Biochemistry of Schizophrenia

Schizophrenia is an old disease with a relatively new name. The disease referred to most frequently as dementia praecox in the nineteenth century is called schizophrenia in the twentieth century. The schism the word alludes to is between the person and reality. Schizophrenic patients have in common an inability to relate to reality the way the majority of people in the population do, but their specific symptoms are highly variable. Most schizophrenics can neither work nor form personal relationships. There has never been an unambiguous line of demarcation, however, between schizophrenics and patients with other psychiatric disorders. Schizophrenia and related diseases have existed throughout history and currently are found in about 1 percent of the U.S. population. The prevalence is similar in all populations and cultures.

Schizophrenia is increasingly thought of as being multiple disease processes. It is possible to make an analogy with cancer. Cancer was at one time considered to be a single disease, or at least the word "cancer," as commonly used in diagnoses, implied one disease. Cancer is now subdivided into a very large number of separate disorders. The diagnosis of schizophrenia may move in the same direction, becoming divided into a host of subcategories, each with a significantly different etiology.

Part of the heterogeneity of the disease may result from what can be called a "spectrum" effect. This is the concept that a single, underlying process, such as an excessive activity of dopamine in the case of schizophrenia, can produce a wide spectrum of apparently different diseases in different people. The diversity in the spectrum is due to differences in the amount of the effect and in differences in the interaction between the single underlying mechanism and other processes, including other diseases, in the person. In the simplest possible spectrum, a single gene mutation, appearing in different degrees in different individuals, could present as a wide range of different, but possibly related, symptoms in genetic relatives. These might be diagnosed as different diseases. Genetic studies of psychiatric illness often find this sort of phenomenon. The primary disease being studied may appear more frequently in biological relatives of patients, but other, possibly related diseases also appear at increased frequency. It is possible that these other diseases may be part of the spectrum of biological expression of a single underlying chemical mechanism.

Schizophrenia is now subdivided to some degree. Many subtypes of schizophrenia are officially recognized and diagnosed, based on differences in the patterns of the various signs and symptoms of the disease. In addition, it is useful to separate the symptoms into two broad categories, negative and positive. Negative symptoms, ranging from social withdrawal to catatonia, correlate to some degree with brain damage. For example, many patients with predominantly negative symptoms have been shown to have enlarged **ventricles** (a system of cavities within the brain that contain CSF and where some of the CSF is produced). Positive schizophrenic symptoms include hallucinations (often auditory) and agitation. The presence of these distinct symptom categories is already indicative of considerable heterogeneity within the diagnosis.

There has been debate about the cause(s) of schizophrenia for as long as it has been recognized. Theories to explain its origin and treatment are both numerous and diverse. Whether the disease was "psychological" or "biological" in origin was a debate that lasted for many years. Much of this debate antedates current understanding that psychological events have molecular and physiological correlates within the brain. Some earlier proposals entirely ruled out a role for physical factors in the schizophrenic disease process. This is currently an unpopular view.

A major shift in opinion about the role of biological factors in schizophrenia came about as a result of genetic studies. There has been some evidence for a genetic role in schizophrenia for at least fifty years, but there was also considerable controversy about the evidence. In the late 1960s the results of a study of schizophrenia in adoptees, using records in Denmark, were published. This study, involving scientists from several countries, examined the historical and medical records of several thousand adoptees. The study, combined with other data, indicated a role for both environmental and genetic factors in the development of schizophrenia. Adoption records clearly showed that schizophrenia was far more common in the adopted children of schizophrenic biological parents than in the adopted children of normal biological parents. The statistics also clearly reveal that schizophrenia is not as strongly hereditary as other biological traits such as eye color or height. Having schizophrenic parents greatly increases one's chances of being diagnosed schizophrenic, at some time in one's life, but does not make it certain.

An identical twin of a schizophrenic has the greatest statistical risk of developing the disease, greater than 50 percent. This is both a high risk, higher than any other identified, and a low risk, in the sense that it is not 100 percent. This finding illustrates that both genetics and environment are etiologic factors in schizophrenia.

The genetic data, when coupled with the efficacy of the drug treatments for schizophrenia that first became available in the 1950s, persuaded most observers that biological (i.e., chemical) factors were important in this disease. If a syndrome is in part genetic in origin, that part must be chemical in nature, since genes (DNA) are chemical. If the syndrome responds to chemical intervention, a chemical imbalance must have been present. This is the current view.

INTERACTION OF GENETICS AND ENVIRONMENT IN THE BRAIN

The interaction of genetics and environment in the brain was touched on in Chapter 12. It is now known that the brain is continuously changing, anatomically and chemically. Changes occur with learning as well as in response to other environmental factors, such as injury. Whenever one group of neurons loses its communications with a second group of neurons, other cells take the opportunity to make connections for themselves. This kind of aggressive synaptic colonization is continuous, possibly throughout life. Therefore, any significant change in environmental influences on the brain is expressed in corresponding physical and chemical changes. An important implication for medicine is that interventions that result in clinical improvements are possible. Diseases with the strongest genetic component may in theory eventually be treatable. This remarkable plasticity of the brain, increasingly a focus of research, provides hope for some treatment of even the most severe diseases.

GENETIC DETERMINANTS OF SCHIZOPHRENIA

Before probing further into biochemical theories of schizophrenia, it is necessary to discuss patterns of genetic determination of the disease. Many diseases are caused by a change (mutation) in a single gene. For example, the lack of the correct gene for a particular beta-hexosaminidase results in Tay-Sachs disease (Chapter 2).

Other diseases are caused by a complex pattern of altered genes. For example, adult-onset diabetes (called type II diabetes) may be caused by several genes working in concert to produce obesity and insulin resistance. Such a disease is referred to as **polygenic,** since it takes multiple genetic alterations in the same organism to produce the disease.

Other disease processes, although referred to as a single disease, can arise from a variety of causes. For example, one person may have gout because of a deficiency of an enzyme that salvages purines (a single mutation in the gene for hypoxanthine-guanine phosphoribosyl transferase [HPRT] creates severe gout in the affected person). Another person with gout may have an increased amount of phosphoribosyl pyrophosphate (PRPP) synthetase, an entirely different mutation. A third person may have gout from an inability of the kidney to excrete uric acid, and so on. When one syndrome can be produced by many different mechanisms, it is referred to as **polygenetic** (not to be confused with polygenic).

For many years schizophrenia was assumed to be polygenic. Because of its complex nature, its different manifestations, and the somewhat ambiguous effects on the mind, it seemed reasonable to assume that alterations in many genes have an additive effect that resulted in the clinical entity called schizophrenia. Considerable data from recent research, however, call this assumption into question. Some of these data also suggest that schizophrenia may be polygenetic. Using a statistical biological technique called genetic linkage analysis, it is possible to analyze the genetic pedigree of a family with a high incidence of schizophrenia. This technique has been used to study multiple afflicted families; each study suggested that a single gene on a particular chromosome was involved. One such study resulted in a focus on a particular part of chromosome 5 (possibly only a single gene on this chromosome). Using essentially the same techniques, other investigators implicated different chromosomes and different genes. The data in one such study implicated a dominant gene with only partial penetrance; another implicated a recessive gene. One could conclude that one or more of these studies is flawed. Another possible conclusion is that schizophrenia is polygenetic in nature. The latter theory is at least biochemically and biologically plausible.

BIOLOGICAL THEORIES OF SCHIZOPHRENIA

Viral Mechanisms

There are several different theories that fit all or part of the genetic and epidemiological data. A virus, for example, could account both for a genetic susceptibility and for the familial nature of the disease. Since viruses attach themselves to specific kinds of chemical sites (or receptors) in the host, people could have a genetic makeup that renders them either susceptible or resistant to a particular virus.

Adoption data somewhat contradict the viral theory, however. Although this theory remains a possibility, viruses as a cause of schizophrenia have not received much attention in recent years.

Autoimmune Mechanisms

As discussed in connection with multiple sclerosis (Chapter 1), the CNS is especially vulnerable to attack by the individual's own immune system because of the blood–brain barrier. Once this barrier has formed in childhood, usually by the age of two, the immune system no longer keeps nervous tissue under continuous surveillance. As a result, antigenic sites (epitopes) that develop after that time will be seen as foreign antigens by the person's own immune system. If the blood–brain barrier is disrupted, the possibility of autoimmunization arises. It is not certain exactly what circumstances set autoimmune disease in motion. A physical disruption of the blood–brain barrier, such as occurs in head injury, can initiate an autoimmune sequence of events and produce symptoms months or years later. A virus infection can disrupt the blood–brain barrier by many mechanisms, including physical disruption, inflammation, and fever. Once autoimmunization has occurred, the immune attack can take place at a later time, despite the presence of the intact barrier. By whatever mechanism, autoimmune diseases often arise weeks to months following a virus infection. In the context of schizophrenia, these observations serve as a bridge between the viral and autoimmune theories of its **etiology.**

Evidence for an autoimmune etiology of schizophrenia includes data indicating that numerous antibodies are found bound to parts of schizophrenics' brains. Given the importance of plasma membrane molecules in brain function, the binding of antibodies to some of them could produce marked mental symptoms. In vitro experiments with antibodies, however, indicate that predicting the effects of such binding will be difficult.

Antibodies to the nicotinic acetylcholine receptor bind to the receptor and inhibit the activity of Ach. Therefore, many of the symptoms of myasthenia gravis, a disease caused by antibodies bound to the nicotinic receptor, are explained by decreased Ach function. On the other hand, antibodies to the receptors for some peptide hormones, such as insulin, have been found to be agonists. These antibodies bind the receptor and are capable of producing the symptoms of an excess of the natural effector. By either mechanism, the autoimmune attack markedly disturbs normal function.

BIOCHEMICAL THEORIES OF SCHIZOPHRENIA

Biochemical theories of the etiology of schizophrenia fit the epidemiological data well. Many such theories have been published over the years, implicating essentially all neurotransmitters, many other regulatory molecules, and many toxins and drugs. Many of these experiments, however, have not been adequately reproduced, despite considerable publicity and many attempts to repeat them. A few hypotheses that have been supported by more than one group of investigators are mentioned here. The major biochemical theory, at present and for the last twenty years, involves the neurotransmitter dopamine. This latter theory is discussed in most detail.

Wheat Gluten

One hypothesis, which lacks a plausible mechanism, is based on gluten, the major protein of wheat. Gluten is widely consumed throughout the world, though not universally. There may be a correlation between rates of schizophrenia and the consumption of wheat products, on a national or international basis.

Several controlled studies of this theory have involved people who were already institutionalized for mental illness. These studies, therefore, do not address the origin and development of the disease, only its exacerbation in people known to be susceptible. In these experiments, the effects of high carbohydrate foods in the diet were studied. Pasta made with wheat flour was provided for one group of patients, and potatoes were provided for another group. The results of these experiments are interesting in that the group that consumed wheat required more time on locked wards. Therefore, there may be a relationship between wheat intake and the worsening of symptoms. Similar experiments have narrowed the focus of attention to the major protein fraction of the wheat, called gluten. The gluten fraction has not been well characterized biochemically, and not much more can be said about these experiments.

Methionine

Another puzzling observation, which has been reproduced by several groups of investigators, involves an infusion of the amino acid methionine into the blood of schizophrenics. This was observed to exacerbate their symptoms. Methionine enters the CNS by the LNAA transporter (Chapter 6), which suggests one of two possible mechanisms as an etiology for the observed effect: either too much methionine or too little of one of the other amino acids substrates for the LNAA. The LNAA transports several amino acids, all of which are essential to normal CNS metabolism. Each substrate amino acid essentially competes with the others for transport, and an excess of one will displace the others. Both tryosine and tryptophan, from which serotonin and the catecholamine neurotransmitters are made, are also substrates for the LNAA. The ability of methionine to exacerbate the symptoms of schizophrenia could be related to a deficiency of one of these transmitters. It is also possible that excess methionine produces the exacerbation of symptoms.

Specific mechanisms by which excess methionine interferes with brain biochemistry are not clear, but two possibilities have been suggested. Each of these links the methionine treatment to other biochemical theories of schizophrenia. Many neurotransmitters are catabolized by having methyl groups added to their structures. Both dopamine and norepinephrine are methylated in synapses, and serotonin is methylated in the process of becoming melatonin. Norepinephrine is also methylated (by a different enzyme) when it is converted to epinephrine. Finally, histamine (a transmitter in the CNS that is not discussed here) is methylated before it is removed from the CNS. The source of the methyl groups in each of these cases is S-adenosyl methionine (SAM). Although the explanation is highly speculative, it is possible that the concentrations of SAM and its precursor, methionine, could be determining factors in this metabolism, and that methylated metabolites, in excess, could disrupt mental function. It may also be relevant that many hallucinogenic molecules are methylated derivatives of these neurotransmitters. Other reactions important in CNS function require SAM. For example, there have been reports of enzymes in synaptic plasma membranes that use SAM to change the structure of lipids within the membrane, and thereby change the fluidity and the receptor interactions of the membrane as well. This also could result in changes in mental function.

The above biochemical hypotheses of schizophrenia, in addition to many others for which some published evidence exists, are fertile areas for future research. Several of the above hypotheses, it should be noted, address only the worsening of symptoms in previously diagnosed schizophrenics. Only the autoimmune hypothesis (and its corollary involving virus infection) addresses the issue of etiology.

NEUROTRANSMITTERS AND SCHIZOPHRENIA

For many years, the major biochemical hypothesis for the etiology of schizophrenia has focused on excessive activity of dopamine (DA). Other, similar theories have focused on norepinephrine and serotonin, but the dopamine hypothesis has remained preeminent. The majority of the evidence for the DA hypothesis is pharmacological, although there are supporting data from direct measurements of DA receptors.

The first major bit of evidence that led to this hypothesis was the discovery of antipsychotic drugs, called neuroleptics. Since they were first developed in the 1950s, there have been several generations of such relatively specific antipsychotic agents. Most of these drugs share the ability to block dopamine receptors. This DA receptor binding has been observed in the brains of autopsied patients, as well as in experimental animals. It has also been observed that the clinical efficacy of antipsychotic drug treatment is, for the most part, directly proportional to the drug's ability to block DA receptors.

In addition to the neuroleptics, drugs that decrease DA activity by other means also alleviate psychotic symptoms. Reserpine (Chapter 6), which functions presynaptically and after a time reduces DA release, is twice as effective as placebos in treating schizophrenia. Drugs that inhibit the synthesis of DA, if given with neuroleptics, decrease the required dose of the receptor blockers. Conversely, drugs that increase dopamine release or activity will worsen psychotic symptoms. For example, amphetamines, long known to increase DA and noradrenaline action, can produce a schizophrenia-like syndrome in previously unaffected people. Other drugs that are agonists for DA receptors can cause psychotic symptoms. One striking bit of evidence of this sort came from observations of patients with Parkinson's disease. These patients suffer from a loss of cells in the major dopaminergic tract in the CNS, the nigrostriatal tract. A treatment for Parkinson's is to administer L-dihydroxyphenylalanine (L-DOPA, or levodopa). L-DOPA can be transported by the LNAA and thereby enter the CNS. DOPA is an intermediate in the synthesis of the catecholamine neurotransmitters, and it occurs in the synthetic pathway after the allosteric enzyme subject to negative feedback control. Therefore, after entering the CNS, DOPA enters cells and is converted into dopamine in any cell that contains aromatic amino acid decarboxylase (AAAD), the final enzyme in dopamine synthesis (Chapter 6). Many cells contain this enzyme, including the remaining dopaminergic cells in Parkinson's patients. Through the action of AAAD, each dopaminergic cell greatly increases the amount of dopamine it releases into the receptive field around its synaptic terminals. This effect is beneficial to many Parkinson's patients. However, about 15 percent of Parkinson's patients treated in this way develop psychotic symptoms resembling those of schizophrenia.

Other cells with AAAD are present in the CNS. They can also increase their production of DA. This is true of noradrenergic cells, serotonergic cells, and others. When such cells increase DA production, DA becomes a "false transmitter," because it is made and released from cells that do not normally use it. In addition, increased DA is synthesized and released from other dopaminergic cells, outside the pathway affected in Parkinson's disease. The two major groups of such DA cells are designated A9 and A10; these groups form the mesolimbic and mesocortical pathways. These nuclei also release extra DA when they obtain administered DOPA. Excessive release of DA from these tracts is thought to be the cause of many of the positive symptoms of schizophrenia and, therefore, is the explanation of the 15 percent of Parkinson's patients on DOPA who show psychotic symptoms.

The above evidence, from several different kinds of pharmacological approaches in humans, supports the dopamine hypothesis of schizophrenia. There is additional support from data in experimental animals. Certain kinds of behaviors in rats are considered models for human psychotic behavior. In particular, a kind of aimless, agitated, searching behavior, called stereotypy, is used as such a model. Stereotypy is drug-induced, and it is increased by treatment with amphetamines and DOPA, both of which increase DA activity. Stereotypy is decreased by treatments that reduce DA activity, including treatment with neuroleptics and even the removal of dopaminergic cells from the brain.

An implication of the dopamine hypothesis is that there should be an increased turnover of DA in schizophrenics, at least in a subset of these patients who are experiencing periods of positive symptoms. If this is so, homovanillic acid (HVA), the catabolic end product of dopamine, should be increased in the CSF of schizophrenics and should likely be even higher during hallucinations or periods of agitation. In fact, HVA has been found to be higher in the CSF of schizophrenics than in normal subjects. At autopsy, these patients also have higher levels of DA and HVA in the mesocortical and mesolimbic tracts.

Since DA is not found in large quantity outside the CNS, the levels of HVA and DA in blood should correlate with dopaminergic activity in brain. In fact, plasma HVA has been found to be higher in untreated schizophrenics than in normal subjects, and it is reduced after treatment with neuroleptics; the length of time it takes for levels to decline matches the diminution of schizophrenic symptoms. Withdrawal from the drug therapy causes a restoration of blood HVA to the levels observed prior to the drug therapy.

Despite the above specifics, levels of HVA in the CSF do not generally correspond well with psychotic symptoms. One possible reason for this is the fact that the majority of DA in the human CNS is not in the mesolimbic and mesocortical tracts, but in the neurons of the substantia nigra, and is released from the nigrostriatal tract. Therefore, alterations of CSF levels of DA and its metabolites correspond better to movement disorders, such as Parkinson's disease, than to **psychosis.**

If the dopamine theory of schizophrenia is correct, or partly correct, many questions remain as to how excessive dopaminergic activity, in the relatively small number of axons in the mesolimbic and mesocortical systems, could cause the signs and symptoms of the disease. These correlations are far from clear despite the enormous advances that have been made. It is possible now to make only some preliminary suggestions. For example, one common symptom of schizophrenia is auditory hallucinations. It has been shown that the brain's auditory system is innervated by the mesolimbic and mesocortical tracts. Therefore, it seems reasonable that increased dopaminergic activity in these tracts could be a partial explanation of the symptom. But there still is no chemical theory about the content of the hallucinations, which may be the most troubling part of the symptom for the afflicted person. Although a genetic and biochemical theory of increased dopaminergic activity may point to a likely therapy (i.e., dopamine antagonists), it does not really "explain" the symptom.

It may be of greater importance that the mesolimbic and mesocortical systems are known to constitute a pleasure center, and schizophrenics are often described as having disordered perceptions of pleasure and pain. Although these facts point to a possible link of a symptom and a pathway, it is still not clear how elevated dopaminergic activity in these tracts could produce the kinds of disorders that are seen in the disease. As mentioned earlier (Chapter 13), some people voluntarily take drugs such as cocaine and/or amphetamines that stimulate this dopaminergic pleasure center. Is it plausible that they are trying to make themselves schizophrenic? Many of them develop symptoms similar to schizophrenia, but this is not usually seen as the person's goal. The actual nature of the defect(s) in schizophrenia is undoubtedly far more complex than a simple hypothesis of "more" or "less" activity of a particular group of neurons. The fundamental mechanisms are much more likely to lie in the (currently unknown) complex systems that regulate these neurons' actions and interactions with the rest of the CNS. Regulatory mechanisms are not usually based on simple changes in the concentration of one or more gene products, but in the interactions of several gene products. The discovery of the details of these interactions is still many years in the future. Final explanations may be partly biochemical, but will require far more research in the fields of psychology, genetics, and biochemistry.

Schizophrenia is a chronic disease. It typically develops during puberty and often persists, off and on, throughout life. Similarly, the therapy for schizophrenia is often administered chronically. Since most of the drugs in current use are blockers of a major dopamine receptor (D2), a chronic blockade of these receptors introduces the problem of the regulatory response. (One of the serotonin receptors, 5HT2, is also implicated.) The postsynaptic cells are not receiving baseline transmitter activity in the presence of the drug. In this case, as is true with the chronic administration of any receptor-binding drug, the system may respond homeostatically. The response is to increase the number of receptors at the postsynaptic sites. This compensatory response in D_2 receptors is believed to be the explanation for the syndrome called tardive dyskinesia.

People afflicted with tardive dyskinesia have uncontrollable, involuntary movements, especially noticeable in the face; they often exhibit mouth and facial muscle twitches of various kinds. This syndrome typically develops only after years of DA receptor blockade therapy, but often it is not reversible by drug withdrawal. It is possible that such long-term changes in receptor number become permanent.

POLYGENESIS

Schizophrenia is possibly a polygenetic disease. The data presented above, in addition to results from many other studies, indicate that increased dopaminergic activity plays an etiologic role in schizophrenia. Other data indicate that this is particularly true of the DA in the mesolimbic and mesocortical pathways, in which dopamine affects parts of the brain known to be involved in higher mentation and emotions. These are the functions most disturbed in schizophrenia. Even if the dopamine hypothesis were correct, and even if it were the only explanation for schizophrenia, schizophrenia could, theoretically, still be a polygenetic disease. Increased DA expression in the mesocortical and mesolimbic tracts can be caused in many different ways. For example, a mutation that reduced the NFB inhibition of tyrosine hydroxylase, the most important regulatory enzyme in the synthesis of DA, would increase the amount of DA made. This, in turn, would lead to increased DA expression from terminals and to increased DA activity at the synapse. A different mutation that led to a greater number of DA receptors, without any change in DA levels, would produce a similar effect. In fact, solely within the dopaminergic synapse, a large number of completely different mutations could cause increased activity or efficacy of dopaminergic synapses.

Mutations affecting the neurons that innervate dopaminergic cells could have similar effects. For example, if glutamate is a stimulator of DA neurons, then a mutation that increased glutamate activity on A9 and A10 sites could produce excess release of DA. Conversely, if GABA is a major inhibitor of DA cells, then a mutation that resulted in decreased GABA activity on mesolimbic DA cells would cause increased release of DA and dopaminergic symptoms. All of these mutations, in the genes for many different molecules and even in different cells, could produce a similar result, an increase in dopaminergic activity in the suspected tracts.

Therefore, even if schizophrenia were caused by a modification of activity of a single transmitter, it could still be a polygenetic disease. Indeed, most diseases, if not all, are likely to be polygenetic to some degree.

SELF-STUDY QUESTIONS

Facts:

1. Which nuclei are dopaminergic?

2. Which parts of the brain do A9 and A10 innervate?

3. What experimental or clinical data lead to the dopamine hypothesis of schizophrenia?

Concepts:

1. Define polygenic.

2. Define polygenetic.

3. Explain the concept of "false transmitters."

4. Discuss how different family pedigrees for schizophrenia could involve different genes and different chromosomes.

BIBLIOGRAPHY

Bellak, L., ed. 1979. *Disorders of the Schizophrenic Syndrome*. New York: Basic Books.

Hemmings, G., ed. 1980. *Biochemistry of Schizophrenia and Addiction*. Baltimore, MD: University Park Press.

Snyder, S.H. 1980. *Biological Aspects of Mental Disorder*. New York: Oxford University Press.

CHAPTER 17

Anxiety and Mood Disorders

Disorders involving anxiety and alterations of mood are among the most frequent causes of visits to physicians. Figures from different studies vary, but a conservative overall estimate is that about 10 percent of the population is likely to seek treatment for one of these disorders in their lifetime. The anxiety syndromes include panic and generalized anxiety, and the affective, or mood, disorders include mania, depression, and manic-depressive disorders. These two categories of mental imbalance, anxiety syndromes and mood disorders, are regarded as separate diagnostic categories, but there is considerable overlap (called comorbidity), with many patients exhibiting aspects of both classes of disease.

In addition to the complexity introduced by comorbidity, there is possibly a "spectrum" effect in both classes of illness. The concept of a spectrum of symptoms was discussed in Chapter 16 in conjunction with schizophrenia, and may also apply to both categories of diseases discussed here. The basic concept is that a single chemical process can produce a wide range of apparently different diseases in different people. This spectrum is due to quantitative differences in the root chemical disorder, differences in the interaction between a genetic predisposition and widely varying life experiences, and differences in the interaction of the predisposition and other parts of the genome. As a result, even in the simplest case, a single gene can produce widely varying symptoms.

As a further complicating factor, disorders of mood and feeling can arise in any person, regardless of genetic predisposition, given sufficient stimulus from the environment. Some people are clearly genetically predisposed to depression and experience it periodically throughout their lifetimes, often with no apparent external cause. Many relatives of these depressives have the same or similar spectrum disorders. Yet anyone can become depressed, and severely so, in response to life experiences—for example, a great loss such as the death of a loved one. Despite the different origin of the symptoms in two such situations, it is quite possible that the depressive feelings themselves are being generated by similar neurotransmitters at similar synapses. In one case the synapses are activated from internal sources; in the other they are activated by external events and the person's internal reaction to them. These distinctions are made even more difficult to study in patients with comorbidity, since depression is a common reaction in otherwise non-depressed people to the development of a serious disease of another kind. All these considerations make it very difficult to study depression in a clear-cut manner.

POSSIBLE BIOLOGICAL MECHANISMS

Several aspects of the pharmacology and biochemistry of anxiety and mood disorders are similar and thus suggest a possible common underlying mechanism. Some of these similarities focus on the locus ceruleus (LC) (see Chapter 6). The LC is noradrenergic, and nearly all the noradrenaline (NE) in the CNS is made and released from its cells. Although the number of noradrenergic synapses in any one part of the brain may be small, the LC innervates much of the CNS. Therefore, although NE is highly centralized in one sense, it has widespread, nearly global, effects, and is important in determining many behavioral and psychological phenomena. The full details of the function and regulation of the LC are not known, but some implications about its function arise from studying the diseases of mood. The following discussion serves as a brief introduction to this highly complex but important structure, and to its possible role in anxiety and mood disorders.

The locus ceruleus has been discussed before (Chapters 6 and 13), and its role as a pleasure center has been mentioned. Pleasure centers were discovered by implanting electrodes in different regions of rats' brains. The rats were then given the opportunity to control stimulation of the electrodes. The areas that the rats stimulated as much as possible, ignoring all other aspects of their environment until they died, were designated "pleasure centers." The LC is a prominent pleasure center, as are the dopaminergic areas that give rise to the mesolimbic and mesocortical systems.

In this light, it is not surprising that people often choose to consume drugs that affect the LC, and that such drugs are often abused. Common psychotropic drugs ranging from alcohol to opiates have potent effects on the LC, but most are *inhibitors*, not stimulators. This raises a question: If the stimulation of the LC produces pleasure, why is there a strong desire (at least in some people) to inhibit it? This question is made more cogent by the observation that the experimental stimulation of an electrode implanted in the LC of a monkey does *not* appear to induce pleasure. The major effect of this stimulation in experimental animals appears to be anxiety. The stimulated animal is agitated, appears fearful, and exhibits the increases in autonomic functions associated with anxiety: blood pressure rises, heart rate and respiration increase, perspiration increases, and so on. Thus, stimulation of the LC (and thereby increasing the release of NE in many parts of the CNS) produces what appears to be a negative experience, and drugs that inhibit this activity may cause experiences that are interpreted as pleasurable by many. These phenomena seem paradoxical: Animals desire self-stimulation of the LC, but its experimental activation appears to cause discomfort and its inhibition may be desirable.

One interpretation of these seemingly paradoxical observations is that what is desirable about self-stimulation of the LC is not the stimulation itself, but its discontinuation. The pleasurable part of the experience may be a kinetic phenomenon, neither stimulation nor inhibition of the LC per se, but the movement from the stimulation to a lack of it. Pleasure may be experienced as a relief from high levels of LC activity, as the activity is associated with anxiety. Simple inhibition of the LC (i.e., when it is not highly activated) can then be interpreted as an avoidance of anxiety, but might not have the actual pleasurable experience associated with relief from anxiety. Although other interpretations are possible, this view is consistent with many of the observations discussed below. In both anxiety and mood disorders, increased NE may be associated with at least a part of the anxious, unpleasant experience, and inhibition of its function may be the mechanism of treatment. Therefore, the same transmitter system could be involved in both pleasure and anxiety.

Seen in this context, it is much more difficult to explain the voluntary use of drugs that stimulate the LC. Are such people deliberately inducing an anxious state in order to escape from it later, or is the direct stimulation of the LC actually directly pleasurable, despite the observations in monkeys? Perhaps different individuals respond differently to such stimulation. It is not yet possible to bring all these observations together with one explanation.

ANXIETY DISORDERS

Anxiety is defined as an "inappropriate level of fear or apprehension for the particular situation." This is different from normal fear, which is an appropriate response to a genuine threat. The somatic symptoms of anxiety include manifestations of elevated sympathetic activity, such as increased heart rate (tachycardia) and breathing (tachypnea), trembling, sweating (diaphoresis), and vasomotor effects (e.g., cold extremities). Anxiety disorders can be clinically subdivided into two broad categories based on pharmacological and genetic criteria: generalized anxiety and panic.

Generalized Anxiety

Generalized anxiety, as a separate psychiatric disease, consists of persistent anxiety without the panic attacks or phobias that are part of other illnesses. The distinction between "normal" anxiety and the official psychiatric diagnosis may not be very clear. The most frequently used drugs for the treatment of generalized anxiety are benzodiazepines, which indicates a likely role for GABA or other amino acid transmitters in the origin of the symptoms (Chapter 4). As discussed earlier, the overall ratio of excitatory to inhibitory amino acid transmitters could be considered as setting the tone of the nervous system. A high ratio creates excitability or irritability; a lower ratio establishes tranquilization. It is possible to think of this amino acid balance as being a kind of "filter" for sensory input, allowing more or less stimulation into the CNS. This concept is based heavily on the fact that the most common therapies for anxiety act upon the GABA-A receptor, increasing GABA's potency as an inhibitor of CNS function.

Amino acid transmitters are globally present and active within the CNS. Besides setting the overall excitation/inhibition tone, they are fundamental to the operation of second- and third-level transmitters. Therefore, any function that is predominantly regulated by, for example, catecholamines would also be affected by amino acid transmitters. If catecholamines generate a disease process from increased synaptic activity, that process can be counteracted either by decreasing the effect of the catecholamines themselves or by modifying the postsynaptic cells in some other way. The effects of the NE released from the LC are superimposed upon the effects of amino acid transmitters. Increasing the inhibitory amino acid input from postsynaptic cells could achieve the same result. Therefore, since most neurons are affected by amino acid transmitters, a disease caused by catecholamines could be treated by using drugs that affect amino acids' receptors. Amino acids likely affect all the cells that respond to NE, as well as the cells that release NE (the LC).

There is minimal evidence for a genetic component of generalized anxiety, although drug treatment with benzodiazepines (BZPs) is most commonly prescribed. BZPs bind to specific binding sites on the GABA-A receptor, as discussed in Chapter 9. These BZP sites are at different subunit locations from those that bind GABA, and they act as positive allosteric modifiers of GABA (i.e., their effect is to increase the GABA effect). Like other well-studied ion channel receptors, the GABA receptor normally has several different allosteric states: resting (R), active (A), and desensitized (D). The acute effect of BZPs is to increase the number of receptor molecules in the A state (which increases the frequency of channel opening). This possibly results from the lowering of the K_D for GABA at its binding site. BZPs also decrease the fraction of receptors in the D state (desensitized by phosphorylation).

When BZPs are consumed chronically, the person develops a tolerance to their sedative and anticonvulsant effects. This is a common, homeostatic response to the long-term presence of synaptically active molecules (Chapter 13). It is possible, however, that a similar tolerance does not develop to the anxiolytic (anxiety-reducing) effects of BZPs. If this is indeed true, their clinical usefulness would remain high even with chronic use. Receptor down regulation is a common response to the chronic use of any agonist, but this secondary allosteric response may not produce a sufficiently strong effect on the receptor to elicit homeostatic down regulation. If this is the case, the question of why patients develop a tolerance to the anticonvulsant and sedative effects of BZPs remains unanswered. With continued usage of benzodiazepines, however, some people tend to become addicted. Addiction occurs in only a small fraction of the total, but is a serious issue to consider.

Since the discovery of endogenous opiates, it is common to look for endogenous molecules that have properties similar to those of useful drugs. A small (molecular weight of about 11,000) endogenous protein has been discovered that is an antagonist to BZP binding. It appears to bind at the same site as BZPs. This peptide has clinical use in cases of BZP overdose. The normal function of this peptide, called the "anxiety peptide," may be to act as a negative regulator of GABA. There is also a class of drugs (beta-carbolines) that inhibit the GABA system and thereby cause anxiety.

Despite the fact that benzodiazepines are the most commonly prescribed therapy for anxiety disorder, some of the drugs aimed at second-level transmitters are also effective. For example, some antidepressants, paradoxically, can be useful in treating anxiety. These drugs are thought to act in the catecholamines' synapses, and their effectiveness against anxiety is further evidence for the concept that LC activity may be part of the origin of anxious symptoms.

It is harder to explain the fact that a few drugs that work at serotonin's synapses also appear to be effective in treating anxiety, at least some of its symptoms. These are drugs that inhibit serotonin's effects and even stimulate the LC. The seeming paradox of this, and of other clinical observations, will be addressed below.

Panic Disorder

Panic is defined as an inappropriate increase in the level of anxiety that lasts a relatively short period of time (5 minutes to 2 hours) and then spontaneously abates (i.e., the state is self-limiting). The average attack is about twenty minutes.

Theoretically, such an increase in anxiety level could be caused by a second-level transmitter system, such as noradrenaline. In this situation, the second-level biogenic amines could provide an increase of the baseline anxiety set by the amino acids. In fact, noradrenaline and/or dopamine are the transmitters most frequently implicated, based on the activity of the drugs used to treat the disorder clinically.

First-degree relatives (parents, children, and siblings) of patients diagnosed with panic disorder tend to have a higher-than-normal incidence of the same disease. Therefore, there is likely a genetic component to panic. This observation also suggests that panic arises from a mechanism distinct from that of generalized anxiety. Panic disorders are often treated with tricyclic antidepressants (TCAs) and with monoamine oxidase inhibitors (MAOIs), although drugs that affect the GABA-A receptor can also be used. Both TCAs and MAOIs are believed to act in catecholamine and serotonin synapses.

Given these observations, the LC can be hypothesized to mediate panic attacks, as it may also have a role in generalized anxiety. Both the TCAs and the MAOIs affect noradrenaline in the LC, and both increase the availability, and therefore the synaptic effects, of NE at its synapses. TCAs, among other things, inhibit the presynaptic re-uptake of NE, thereby increasing the amount in the synaptic cleft. This, in turn, increases the amount of postsynaptic receptor activation. MAOIs, as the name suggests, inhibit monoamine oxidase (MAO), the enzyme that destroys catecholamines and serotonin in their presynaptic terminals. If MAO cannot function, the amount of NE and serotonin is increased within the cytoplasm of the terminals, then in the synaptic vesicles, and later in the synaptic cleft.

There are a large number of published reports linking anxiety to elevated noradrenaline levels (or at least to increased methoxy hydroxy phenylethyl glycol [MHPG], the final CNS metabolite of noradrenaline). This association is true not only in the case of the anxiety present in the anxiety disorders discussed above, but also in the case of the anxiety found in the mood disorders, discussed next.

MOOD DISORDERS

Because of the well-established efficacy of "biological" treatments for mood disorders, including not only drugs but such interventions as electroconvulsive shock therapy, it is commonly assumed that mood disorders are chemical in origin. Genetic studies tend to support this hypothesis. Mood disorders, also called affective illnesses, are familial, with a much greater concordance among identical twins than fraternal twins. Attempts to find a simple, unifying neurochemical theory of mood disorders have not been particularly successful, however.

There is also a spectrum of diseases involving mood, and an increased incidence of these spectrum disorders (in addition to yet other diseases) in the close biological relatives of affected individuals. The affective diseases are more severe disturbances than anxiety and panic disorders, and they account for a large fraction of psychoses. Mood disorders are usually subdivided into unipolar and bipolar types. Unipolar illness is characterized by depression alone, and bipolar illness is characterized by swings of mood, including depression and manic episodes. Given the complexity of the data and the elusiveness of a unifying hypothesis, it is quite possible that mood disorders are truly polygenic, or that they are both polygenic and polygenetic.

This discussion focuses on only a few of the basic interactions between transmitters and between transmitters and receptors. The transmitters most implicated in mood disorders include those most likely involved in the spectrum of anxiety disorders, as well as others: GABA, dopamine (DA), noradrenaline (NE), and serotonin (5-HT). The focus is again on the LC and the Raphe nucleus, and there are indications of a possible role for dopamine. The brain's pleasure centers are both noradrenergic and dopaminergic; serotonin is a major inhibitor of both systems.

Most published studies linking neurotransmitters with mood disorders focus on catecholamines. Two intriguing observations implicate serotonin, however. Both have been reproduced by different, independent investigators. The first is that serotonin's final CNS metabolite, 5-hydroxyindole acetic acid (5-HIAA) (Chapter 7), is decreased in the CSF of people who commit suicide. The second observation is that, at autopsy, the levels of 5-HT receptors in the brains of suicide victims are increased. These facts can be interpreted as indicating that suicidally depressed people have either too much or too little serotonin activity. That is, either they have too many 5-HT receptors, causing a depression from too much activity, or they produce and express too little serotonin, causing depression. In either case, these observations can be seen as the brain's attempt to compensate for the primary imbalance. Either the brain of the person with too many receptors tries to compensate by decreasing the 5-HT production, or the brain of the person with too little 5-HT increases receptor number. An additional observation is relevant. There are reports that serotonin function is diminished in many people who commit murder, or are guilty of other highly impulsive, dangerous behaviors. One interpretation that summarizes all the above data is that decreased serotonin function is associated with less psychic inhibition, or self-control, and therefore with violent behavior. Whether the person turns the violence against self (as in depression, to the extreme of suicide) or others (as in violent aggression, to the extreme of murder) is determined by other factors. This hypothesis would focus on too little serotonin as being a causative factor in either case.

Another reproduced observation links MHPG, the final CNS catabolite of NE, to anxiety, as mentioned above. This link has been observed in cases of anxiety from different diagnostic categories. Putting this observation together with the above data, and the fact that 5-HT is an important inhibitor of the LC, allows the following conjectures. Diminished serotonin may be associated with impulsive, sometimes violent, behavior, and this behavior possibly occurs, at least in part, through the diminution of the inhibition of the LC. Increased NE expression would result from diminished inhibition of the LC, and NE is a potent, widespread transmitter of arousal. Serotonin is also an inhibitor of dopaminergic cells, many of which are involved in motor activity. Decreased serotonin inhibition of these dopaminergic tracts would therefore allow increased physical movement.

If, in some circumstances, LC arousal is negative, as seen in experimental animals, NE would be the more direct cause of anxiety. It is therefore possible that the LC is capable of generating both pleasant arousal and unpleasant arousal (i.e., anxiety) as was seen in the pleasure center studies. The other catecholamine, DA, may cause inappropriate motor activity, and decreased serotonin may result in inappropriately high levels of both catecholamines. Although these preliminary hypotheses are undoubtedly oversimplifications, they provide a basis for developing therapeutic interventions and for further research.

Besides being inhibited by serotonin, the LC is subject to a large amount of self-inhibition, a kind of negative feedback. The cluster of noradrenergic cell bodies that make up the LC sends axons to many other parts of the CNS and also has many axon collaterals that loop back onto it. These autosynapses, containing alpha receptors on the postsynaptic (i.e., perikaryal) membranes, are inhibitory to the LC. Thus, stimulation of the LC produces a stimulation of many other parts of the CNS and simultaneously initiates an autoinhibition. Therefore, the LC is inhibited by noradrenaline, serotonin, and other transmitters, as well as other drugs. It is simultaneously stimulated by other transmitters.

Drug Therapies

One of the most important drug therapies for manic disorders is lithium (Li^+). Li^+ is also effective in some depressive disorders. Since the mechanism of action of effective therapeutic drugs can give insight into the mechanism of a disease, Li^+ has been thoroughly studied. As with many other drugs that affect the CNS, a major difficulty in interpreting the data about lithium's mechanism of action is that it has so many actions. Li^+, because of its size and charge, works in many enzyme systems as an antagonist for Mg^{++}. As Mg^{++} is necessary for all enzymes that hydrolyze triphosphates (i.e., ATP, GTP, etc.), Li^+ also has effects in every metabolic pathway and enzymatic regulatory system. Lithium also inhibits many phosphatases, enzymes that hydrolyze a single phosphate from a substrate. There are a variety of these enzymes, which together have a wide range of substrate specificity.

The Li^+ ion has been shown to bind to G proteins, at or near the site at which GTP binds. It may be of greater importance that this binding interferes with the coupling of the receptor to the G protein. Chapter 11 pointed out that the last intercellular loop of the heptahelical receptor family has multiple regulatory sites, and that this loop is also the site of binding to G proteins. Therefore, lithium's inhibition of this binding serves to decrease the effects of all receptors that use a G protein for their second messenger responses. Thus, Li^+ potentially can affect any receptor in the heptahelical family. It will have a greater effect in biogenic amine and peptide synapses than in amino acid synapses.

Although this insight into Li's mechanism of action focuses attention on one aspect of its binding, it does not completely explain the range of its effects. G proteins are themselves a highly heterogeneous family. If Li^+ had a greater effect on a particular kind of G protein than on others, its mechanism of psychotherapeutic action might become much clearer. At present, it has to be considered as a useful but rather nonspecific drug. Li^+ has so many sites of action that its mechanism does not at present help clarify the basic mechanisms of the diseases for which it is used.

Tricyclic Antidepressants (TCAs) and Monoamine Oxidase Inhibitors (MAOIs).

Many of the drugs used to treat depression are similar to those used in panic disorders, TCAs and MAOIs. Although the two moods are different (perhaps opposite), depression may be accompanied by anxiety. Both of these classes of drugs are known to work in the biogenic amine systems. Other drugs that work in these systems have therapeutic uses in either mania or depression. For example, reserpine, which depletes catecholaminergic and serotonergic terminals of their transmitters, causes a severe depression in some patients. Pharmacological observations such as these originally led to the biogenic amine hypothesis of mood disorders, that is, that deficiencies in the concentrations of some of these transmitters cause depression and elevated concentrations cause mania. The specifics of the hypothesis have not been completely supported by experimental evidence, with the exceptions cited above, despite a very large number of such studies. Some aspects of this hypothesis remain plausible, however, and it is possible that mood disorders originate with a malfunctioning of the biogenic amine transmitter systems. One fundamentally troubling issue, however, is the fact that similar kinds of drugs, such as TCAs and MAOIs, can be useful in treating symptoms like panic and depression that seem to be the opposite of each other. It would seem that the only reasonable interpretation of these facts is that the underlying cause of the disease cannot be merely an overactivity or underactivity of a particular transmitter, but that it must lie in regulatory phenomena—that a mental disease state occurs, not just from too much or too little of a transmitter, but from inappropriate responses of that transmitter to other stimuli.

One fundamental aspect of manic-depressive illness is the time course of symptoms. Therefore, the basic flaws leading to these disorders may not lie simply in the quantity of available transmitters, but in the kinetics of the regulation of their release and function. Regulatory phenomena are too complex to be covered thoroughly in an introductory discussion such as this one. For example, the previous discussions have focused on regulatory events within a single synapse. When considering mood or affect, which are properties of the entire organism, it is necessary at least to take into account the balances between several different transmitter systems, each of which is regulated by other transmitters at all three levels. These transmitters and their receptors are under separate genetic controls. In short, the biochemistry of disorders of affect is not likely to be completely clarified until their neurobiology has been, and that will require a great deal more information. In the meantime, there are some clear indicators that answers may be revealed through the study of NE, 5HT, and DA (and possibly Ach).

Receptor Sensitivity Modification

As mentioned above, mood disorders involve complex temporal phenomena, among other factors. A strong piece of evidence for this conclusion is the fact that drug therapy for these disorders (and others) typically requires weeks before becoming fully effective. These drugs most commonly used to treat mood disorders are often thought of as having short-term synaptic effects. In vitro and in other experimental conditions, these effects can be clearly shown and quantified, and they take effect quickly after being introduced into the synaptic systems involved. Yet the clinical effectiveness may not be observed for weeks after the introduction of the drug. The most likely interpretation of this timing focuses attention on the regulatory mechanisms of synaptic function, as they operate over a period of days, weeks, months, or even longer.

For example, in treating panic attack, one suggested approach is to use the technique called "receptor sensitivity modification." This is a deliberate use of the long-term regulatory systems that may also underlie the development of addiction to some psychotropic drugs. A common response to the chronic presence of a drug is homeostatic and, thus, compensatory in nature. The intervention in receptor sensitivity modification is designed to cause a long-term compensatory response in receptor number. The short-term effect of the drug therapy, however, is in the opposite direction from the one desired in the long term. Therefore, this technique requires a short-term worsening of the patient's symptoms. This aspect of the procedure makes its use highly controversial and often requires hospitalization of the patient. After the initial period of worsening symptoms, a long-term change in receptor number occurs. This change may last for several months without further drug use.

The current use of TCAs for the treatment of panic disorder may be an example of this technique. One theory of the cause of panic disorder is that the patient has an increased number of noradrenergic receptors or an increased receptor sensitivity to NE. This increase could be either genetic or environmental in origin. Nevertheless, when TCAs (or MAOIs) are administered acutely, they increase noradrenergic synaptic activity. This is likely to worsen anxiety. During this acute period, the patient's symptoms may in fact worsen. With chronic use of the drug, however, a down regulation of the NE receptors, in those synapses where NE activity is increased, can be expected. This down regulation would require from several days to weeks to occur. Once the number of receptors is reduced, it may be possible to discontinue the drug. Thus, current practice may already be using the receptor sensitivity modification technique. Obviously, much more data are required before any clear conclusions can be drawn.

SELF-STUDY QUESTIONS

Facts:

1. What is the predominant neurotransmitter believed to be involved in generalized anxiety?

2. Which neurotransmitter is believed to predominate in panic disorders, thus distinguishing these from generalized anxiety?

3. Describe the effect of BZPs on GABA-A receptors.

4. What are the mechanisms of action of TCAs and MAOIs?

Concepts:

1. Discuss the effects of both chronic and acute BZP administration on the GABA–BZP receptor complex.

2. Discuss possible acute and chronic effects of MAOIs and TCAs on LC and Raphe function.

3. Discuss a possible mechanism for the increased LC activity hypothesized to be involved in panic attack.

4. Discuss the possible functions of endogenous anxiogenic molecules.

5. Discuss the mechanisms by which a genetic predisposition for a disease can produce a spectrum of disorders in first degree relatives.

6. Discuss the difference between a disease process caused by a disorder of regulation of transmitter level, as opposed to a disorder just of transmitter level.

BIBLIOGRAPHY

Eichelman, B.S. 1990. Neurochemical and psychopharmacological aspects of aggressive behavior. *Ann. Rev. Medicine* 41:149–158.

Friedhoff, A.J., and Miller, J.C. 1983. Clinical implications of receptor sensitivity modification. *Annual Review of Neuroscience* 6:121–148.

Goodwin, F.K., and Jamison, K.R. 1990. *Manic-Depressive Illness*. New York: Oxford University Press.

Sachar, E.J., and Baron, M. 1979. The biology of affective disorders. *Annual Review of Neuroscience* 2:505–518.

Answers to Self-Study Fact Questions

CHAPTER 1

1. Oligodendrocytes, in the CNS, provide a portion of the myelin sheath to many axons. Schwann cells, in the PNS, provide a portion of the myelin sheath to a single axon. Astrocytes cover the parts of neurons that are not myelinated, including synapses. Microglia (i.e., macrophages) move about within the CNS. Therefore, in the CNS, each glial cell may be close to many neurons, and each neuron may face many glial cells.

2. There are about 10^{11} neurons in the human CNS, and about ten times that number of all glial cells combined. Neurons are, on average, about ten times as large as glial cells. Therefore, about half the total brain substance is glial and about half is neuronal. Neurons and oligodendrocytes are post-mitotic; once they are lost they must be replaced by other cells. Astrocytes are mitotic; they "fill in" the spaces where other cells have died. Neuronal metabolism is normally much higher than that of glial cells, in adults. (Oligodendrocytes have a high metabolic rate in children, when myelin is being made.) Neurons metabolize much faster when they are electrically active. Oxidative rates in the associated astrocytes decrease when the neuronal rate increases.

3. Myelination progresses from the evolutionarily "oldest" parts of the nervous system to the newest: the PNS myelinates first, then the spinal cord, and so on, with the tracts that interconnect different parts of the cortex myelinating last.

4. The major difference between myelinated and unmyelinated axons is the fact that action potentials take place only at the nodes of Ranvier when myelin is present. Myelin has evolutionary utility, first, because it decreases the amount of ATP required for action potentials. This is because the number of Na^+ and K^+ ions that are moved across the axon's membrane decreases during recovery from an action potential. Second, myelin increases the speed at which action potentials are conducted from the cell body to the axon terminal. Third, myelin insulates nearby axons from the electrical current being carried by an axon.

5. Schwann cells, in the PNS, provide only one segment of myelin to one axon. Therefore, one axon has many Schwann cells, but each Schwann cell

has only one neuron. In the CNS, oligodendrocytes contribute a single portion of myelin to as many as fifty or more axons. Therefore, each axon has many glial cells, and each glial cell has many axons.

6. Lipids are molecules that are, for the most part, more soluble in organic solvents such as chloroform or methanol (or their combinations) than in water. Phospholipids are lipids that contain a phosphate residue. Cerebrosides are sphingolipids (i.e., lipids that contain a residue of sphingosine) that contain a single sugar residue, most commonly galactose. Sulfatides are cerebrosides that also have a sulfate residue attached to the sugar (making them more hydrophilic). Cholesterol is a sterol, containing a total of twenty-seven carbons with four fused rings and a "tail" containing eight carbons. A single hydroxyl group is attached to the first ring, giving the molecule a slightly hydrophilic character. All these lipids are found predominantly in membranes.

7. The most prominent autoantigen in myelin is the myelin basic protein (MBP, or simply BP). Other molecules such as proteolipid protein (PLP), gangliosides, and cerebroside also contribute to autoimmunogenicity.

8. Fast anterograde axoplasmic flow uses kinesin as its "motor" and carries formed elements (i.e., neurotransmitter vesicles, membranes, mitochondria, etc.). Fast retrograde flow uses dynein as its motor and carries primarily lysosomes and related structures. Both of these move at a rate of tens to hundreds of millimeters per day. Slow transport component b carries cytoplasmic components and some portions of the cytoskeleton, uses dynamin as its motor, and moves at a few millimeters per day. Slow transport component a moves at less than 1 millimeter per day and carries neurofilaments and neurotubules (the bulk of the cytoskeleton). Both slow components move in the anterograde direction.

CHAPTER 2

1. GM4: NANA-galactose-ceramide

    GM3: NANA-galactose-glucose-ceramide

    GM2: GalNac-galactose-glucose-ceramide
    |
    NANA

    GM1: Galactose-galNac-galactose-glucose-ceramide
    |
    NANA

    GD1a: Galactose-galNac-galactose-glucose-ceramide
    | |
    NANA   NANA

2. All known catabolism of membrane constituents (such as glycosphingolipids) takes place in lysosomes. This catabolism involves simply the hydrolysis of the larger molecules to their component small molecular parts. The bulk of the synthesis of glycoconjugates (i.e., the attachment of sugars both to proteins and to lipids) occurs in the Golgi apparatus.

3. Oligodendrocytes make cerebrosides, sulfatides, and GM4. These molecules are catabolized in these cells, as well. Myelin also contains ganglioside GM1, and it may also be made in oligodendrocytes. Neurons make gangliosides (except for GM4), including the highly complex ones, and neurons also catabolize them. In general, ceramides with a glucose attached to the sphingosine are made neuronally, and those with a galactose attached to the sphingosine are made by oligodendrocytes.

4. a. Sulfatide $\longrightarrow$ cerebroside $\longrightarrow$ ceramide $\longrightarrow$ sphingosine
   b. GM1 $\longrightarrow$ GM2 $\longrightarrow$ GM3 $\longrightarrow$ galactose-glucose-ceramide $\longrightarrow$
      glucose-ceramide $\longrightarrow$ ceramide $\longrightarrow$ sphingosine

5. a. GM1: sialic acid, 2 galactoses, glucose, N-acetyl galactosamine, sphingosine, fatty acid
   b. Sulfatide: sulfate, galactose, sphingosine, fatty acid

6. Tay–Sachs disease: hexosaminidase (a particular isoenzyme)
   Gaucher's disease: a beta glucosidase, sometimes called glucocerebrosidase
   Globoid cell leukodystrophy (GLD): a beta galactosidase
   Metachromatic leukodystrophy (MLD): a sulfatase (a particular isoenzyme)
   Niemann–Pick disease: sphingomyelinase (the enzyme that breaks the ceramide-phosphorylcholine bond)

7. Tay–Sachs disease: ganglioside GM2
   Gaucher's disease: glucocerebroside
   GLD: psychosine (galactose-sphingosine)
   MLD: sulfatide
   Niemann–Pick disease: sphingomyelin (in types A and B)

CHAPTER 3

1. The following types of molecules are found in synaptic vesicles: (a) the transmitter itself; (b) in many cases, a co-transmitter (a peptide is often a co-transmitter with a biogenic amine); (c) ATP; (d) metal ions (often Mg^{++}); (e) a storage glycoprotein; (f) in a few cases, a synthetic enzyme (e.g., dopamine beta hydroxylase in noradrenaline vesicles); (g) co-factors for any synthetic enzymes (vitamin C and Cu^{++} ions in noradrenaline vesicles).

2. Synthesis of small molecule transmitters (i.e., amino acids, biogenic amines) occurs in the cytoplasm, with a few enzymes in vesicles (see above). Synthesis of peptides occurs in the perikaryon of the cell, before the precursors of the transmitters are transported to the axon terminals.

Catabolism of transmitters occurs outside the cell in some cases (e.g., in the case of acetylcholine and peptides) and in the presynaptic terminal in other cases. The catabolism of GABA occurs in astrocytes near the GABA synapses; not much occurs in the neurons themselves. Therefore, synthesis is localized to the neuron that releases the transmitter; catabolism is more variable.

CHAPTER 4

1. Glutamate and aspartate are the main excitatory amino acid transmitters, and GABA and glycine are the major inhibitory transmitters. Both excitatory transmitters have two negative charges on their molecules, whereas the inhibitory transmitters have only one negative charge. All amino acid transmitters have a positive charge, as well. Such putative transmitters as alanine, taurine, and serine would likely be inhibitory. Despite these generalizations, there are special receptors that use these transmitters in exceptional ways. For example, the excitatory NMDA receptor requires glycine in addition to an excitatory amino acid, and there is an inhibitory glutamate receptor in the retina.

2. Most glutamate (excitatory amino acid) receptors open rather non-specific monovalent cation channels. These allow both Na^+ and K^+ ions through, so the major effect of glutamate receptors is excitation due to the entry into the cell of Na^+. The NMDA glutamate receptor is also excitatory, but its opening allows Ca^{++} ions to enter the cell, as well. Both Na^+ and Ca^{++} produce a depolarization, with Ca^{++} producing the greater effect. GABA and glycine both open Cl^- channels, allowing equilibration of the Cl^- concentration across the membrane and thereby making it harder to depolarize or activate the cell. These are therefore inhibitory receptors.

3. Glutamate and glycine are inactivated (i.e., their activity at their postsynaptic receptors is terminated) by re-uptake into the presynaptic terminal. GABA is taken up by nearby glial cells, rather than moving back into the terminal that released it.

CHAPTER 5

1. Ach is synthesized by choline acetyltransferase, abbreviated ChAT or CAT. It requires acetyl CoA and choline as substrates, and its activity is regulated by the choline concentration.

2. The best-known Ach tracts are interneurons (i.e., neurons with short axons that connect two other, nearby neurons), especially those in the spinal cord and in the striatum. Tracts from the nucleus basalis of Meynert, which innervate many parts of the cortex, have also been well studied. Cholinergic cell bodies in the septal area innervate the hippocampus, in a tract thought to be important for learning.

3. The major subclasses of Ach receptors are nicotinic and muscarinic. Both are found outside the CNS, with nicotinic receptors predominant on muscle cells, determining muscles' response to nervous signals. Within the CNS, muscarinic receptors predominate. There are several subtypes of muscarinic receptor, but all use second messengers. Many use the inositol phosphatide system.

4. Ach is hydrolyzed, outside the cell, by the enzyme acetylcholinesterase (AChE).

5. Choline has a relatively specific transporter that takes it back into the presynaptic terminal. There it can be reused for the synthesis of acetylcholine.

6. Ach is stored with a particular storage glycoprotein called vesiculin. The vesicles also contain several other substances, such as ATP and Mg^{++}.

CHAPTER 6

1. In the CNS, the bulk of dopamine (DA) is in the nigral-striatal tract, which extends from the substantia nigra to the neostriatum. There are also two small dopaminergic nuclei (called A9 and A10) near the substantia nigra that send axons to many parts of the cortex and limbic system. These are called the mesolimbic and mesocortical tracts. Almost all the noradrenaline (norepinephrine, NE) in the CNS comes from the cell bodies of the locus ceruleus (LC), which sends axons to much of the rest of the brain.

2. DA is mostly involved in regulation of motor functions. The mesolimbic and mesocortical tracts may be involved in higher cognition. Their functions are not entirely clear. A general increase of DA in the CNS causes greater motor activity of the organism (e.g., more gross motor movement, more sexual activity). NE is primarily involved in psychological arousal, activating the organism to enhanced vigilance and a higher level of attention and awareness. Increasing NE in the CNS causes greater autonomic activity (similar to that observed in connection with anxiety) and greater attention (i.e., enhanced learning).

3. Both DA and NE have multiple receptors, but the most common ones are connected to the cAMP second messenger system. The most common response of postsynaptic cells to receiving DA or NE is inhibition, possibly as the result of an increased K^+ ion permeability.

4. See the answer to question 3, above. The major postsynaptic receptors, D1 (for DA) and beta (for NE), are coupled to adenylyl cyclase, increasing the concentration of cAMP in the postsynaptic cell's cytoplasm. D2 and alpha receptors are often presynaptic and usually lead to decreased cAMP.

5. Synaptic inactivation is by Na^+-coupled re-uptake into the presynaptic terminal.

6. The enzymes that synthesize DA are cytoplasmic. (The final enzyme, aromatic amino acid decarboxylase, may possibly be associated with the cytoplasmic surface of the synaptic vesicles.) The last enzyme in the synthesis of NE is within the synaptic vesicles.

7. Monoamineoxidase (MAO) is on the outer mitochondrial membrane, positioned in such a way that it affects molecules in the cytoplasm. Catechol-O-methyl transferase (COMT) is attached to the plasma membrane of neural cells, in such a way that it affects molecules in the extracellular fluid. Aldehyde reductases and aldehyde oxidases appear to be ubiquitous.

CHAPTER 7

1. An overall increase of serotonin (5-HT) in the CNS produces a generalized decrease in every activity of the organism except sleep. Both total sleep time and total dreaming sleep (REM) time are increased. Generalized motor activity and sexual activity are decreased.

2. There are many subclasses of 5-HT receptors, but the best characterized ones are connected to the inositol phosphate second messenger system. Serotonin therefore tends to be excitatory to its postsynaptic cells.

CHAPTER 8

1. MENK: tyrosine-glycine-glycine-phenylalanine-methionine (abbreviated YGGFM)
LENK: tyrosine-glycine-glycine-phenylalanine-leucine (abbreviated YGGFL)

2. Many enzymes are required. The best known are endopeptidases that cleave peptide bonds containing a basic amino acid (i.e., either lysine, K, or arginine, R). There must also be enzymes that cleave off the basic amino acids, once the precursor peptides have been broken down. In addition, a well-characterized enzyme converts a C-terminal glycine residue to an amide of the penultimate amino acid by oxidizing the two carbons of the glycine to carbon dioxide. This enzyme is called peptidyl glycine alpha-amidating monooxygenase (PAM). The other required enzymes have not yet been well characterized.

3. The messenger RNAs for neuropeptides generally code for proteins that have more than one active neuropeptide within them. Three have been characterized for opioids: proopiomelanocortin (POMC), proenkephalin A, and proenkephalin B (or prodynorphin). The first contains beta endorphin in addition to ACTH, a form of MSH, and other peptides. The second contains multiple MENKs, a LENK, and other related peptides. The last contains multiple active opioid peptides, in several different forms, most of which are either LENK or residues of LENK with extensions on the C terminus. The

first amino acids in the extension are basic ones. Two other well-characterized messenger RNAs are protachykinin and procholecystokinin. The first contains both substance P and substance K; the second contains only derivatives of CCK, the main one of which is CCK-8.

4. Substance P is best known as the "pain peptide," being the transmitter for primary sensory afferents. Its other pathways are in the cerebrum, where it may be involved in the focus of attention. CCK-8 is present at high levels in the cortex (although its function there is unknown). It is also the main transmitter from the paraventricular nucleus (PVN) to the ventral-medial nucleus (VMH) of the hypothalamus. In this tract, it decreases consumption of food by increasing the feeling of satiety. MENK is found in many parts of the CNS but is best characterized as a presynaptic modulator of substance P synapses. In this location, the release of MENK onto the substance P terminus decreases the amount of substance P released, and therefore diminishes the perception of pain.

5. Since the major enzymes of neuropeptide catabolism require free, charged groups at both the N and C termini, neutralizing these two groups increases the peptides' metabolic life. Amidation of the C terminus is described in the answer to question 2, above. There is also at least one enzyme that can attach an acetyl group to the N-terminal amino, using acetyl CoA.

6. Enzymes that degrade neuropeptides include: carboxypeptidases, which remove one C-terminal amino acid; dipeptidyl carboxypeptidases, which remove a C-terminal dipeptide (i.e., two amino acids attached by a single peptide bond); aminopeptidases, which remove a single N-terminal amino acid; and dipeptidyl aminopeptidases, which remove an N-terminal dipeptide.

CHAPTER 9

1. Most amino acid neurotransmitters use direct receptors (i.e., ligand-activated ion channels). The nicotinic acetylcholine receptor is also a direct receptor.

2. Inhibitory postsynaptic potentials (ipsp's) are usually produced by increasing K^+ permeability, increasing Cl^- permeability, decreasing Na^+ permeability, or decreasing Ca^{++} permeability.

3. Excitatory postsynaptic potentials (epsp's) are most commonly produced by increasing Na^+ permeability, increasing Ca^{++} permeability, or decreasing K^+ permeability.

CHAPTER 10

1. Visual receptor cells, of course, are in the eye, specifically, in the last part of the retina to be struck by a photon of light. The photon must therefore pass

through the entire eye, including several layers of cells in the retina, before reaching the visual receptor. Within the receptor cell, the light must pass through the inner segment, containing the nucleus, mitochondria, and other standard cell parts, before arriving at the actual site of phototransduction. In rod cells, transduction occurs in discs, and in cones it takes place in a specialized portion of the plasma membrane. The visual pigments are situated with the site of photon absorption within the relevant membrane, and the several processes of phototransduction occur in the cytoplasm or on the membrane bordering it.

2. In rod cells, rhodopsin absorbs the energy of the photon in its chromophore, cis-retinal. This energy produces changes in the structural conformation of rhodopsin and also results in the cleavage of the retinal group from the protein. The structurally modified (i.e., allosterically activated) rhodopsin binds to, and in turn activates, a G protein. The activated G protein binds to a GTP molecule, which in turn modifies the structure of the G protein, making it an allosteric activator of a phosphodiesterase (PDE). The PDE, when activated, hydrolyzes cGMP. The cGMP is an allosteric activator of a plasma membrane ion channel. While cGMP is bound to the channel, the channel remains open, allowing Na^+ and Ca^{++} ions to enter the cytoplasm of the cell and depolarize the cell. When PDE decreases the concentration of cGMP, the channel closes, resulting in a repolarization (or a hyperpolarization) of the rod cell. When hyperpolarized, the cell secretes less neurotransmitter. Since the transmitter is inhibitory, the net result of the entire sequence is that the absorption of a photon of light results in decreased inhibition of the postsynaptic cell.

3. The means by which rhodopsin is restored is not entirely clear, but one likely process is a light catalyzed restoration of the retinal group back to its 11-cis form. This may occur while the retinal chromophore is attached to a lipid. The restored cis-retinal is then enzymatically returned to an opsin molecule, restoring rhodopsin.

CHAPTER 11

1. Neurotransmitters that use second messenger coupled receptors have different receptors, using multiple systems. Certain generalizations can be made, however. The major postsynaptic receptors for dopamine and noradrenaline are coupled to the cAMP system, commonly increasing cAMP, although they both have secondary receptors that decrease cAMP. The best-studied receptors for acetylcholine and serotonin are coupled to the inositol phosphate system, although these neurotransmitters also have some receptors coupled to cAMP. Peptide transmitters' receptors may be similar in their second messengers to the biogenic amines, although with different kinetics. Some of the more recently discovered "transmitters," such as nitric oxide, use other second messengers, such as cGMP.

2. The best-known second messenger, cAMP, works primarily in the

cytoplasm, although it also has important actions at the genome. Although it is chemically similar to cAMP and also functions in the cytoplasmic compartment, cGMP's functions are less well known. It often binds to the cytoplasmic surface of molecules in the plasma membrane, and it also activates a protein kinase. The inositol phosphate system produces at least two major second messengers: DAG works in the specialized compartment where the cytoplasm and the plasma membrane meet, and IP3 opens a channel allowing Ca^{++} to enter the cytoplasm from the lumen of the endoplasmic reticulum.

3. Protein kinase A (PKA) is activated by cAMP. Its substrates include a wide range of proteins: cytoplasmic enzymes, cytoskeletal proteins, and several proteins that interact with the genome. The functions of cAMP are less well known, but it often binds to an ion channel in the plasma membrane. Diacylglycerol (DAG) binds to and activates protein kinase C (PKC). IP3 binds to a Ca^{++} ion channel. Ca^{++} activates several enzymes by itself, and many others when Ca^{++} is bound to calmodulin.

4. Gs stands for a stimulatory G protein that activates either a phosphodiesterase in the rod cell in the retina or adenylyl cyclase from the cytoplasm. Gi stands for an inhibitory G protein that inhibits adenylyl cyclase from the cytoplasm.

5. NE binds to the receptor, changing its three-dimensional structure. This new structure binds to Gs, activating it to bind to GTP. The Gs, with GTP bound to it, activates adenylyl cyclase, producing an increase in cAMP concentration in the cytoplasm. The cAMP activates protein kinase A, which then phosphorylates a large number of proteins.

CHAPTER 12

1. Learning is the modification of behavior as a result of experience. STM, or short-term learning, is learning that is transient. It has no fixed representation in the brain, disappearing when the organism's attention is turned from it. STM can last, at most, from one sleep period to the next in a human being. LTM, or long-term memory, is learning that is retained for long periods (months or years). It may be permanent. It is, however, capable of being continually modified. Therefore, LTM is not fully stable, although it is long lasting.

2. DNA turnover is unaffected by LTM consolidation, although the expression of some genes is likely increased. New RNA is made and expressed, and protein is made from it. Therefore, both RNA and protein turnover are increased by LTM consolidation. Proteins and lipids of specific types, especially those found in synaptic membranes, are newly synthesized, and therefore also have increased turnover during LTM consolidation.

3. LTM consolidation probably involves the facilitation of synapses in

widespread areas of the brain. Therefore, large parts of the brain are necessary for the storage of memories. Most likely, certain kinds of memories are stored in particular locations. The consolidation process requires at least one hippocampus and one dorso-medial thalamus. Other structures, such as the amygdala and the locus ceruleus, may also be necessary.

4. Potentiation in *Aplysia* requires a facilitating neuron that is serotonergic. Its synapse in this sytem is presynaptic, ending on the synaptic terminal of another neuron, which is in turn synapsing onto a motor cell. When the serotonergic presynaptic synapse is active, cAMP increases postsynaptically (i.e., in the other presynaptic terminal). PKA phosphorylates synaptic proteins such as synapsin (a regulator of synaptic vesicles binding to the plasma membrane), resulting in a delay in the K^+ current of the presynaptic potential. This delay in turn causes an increase in the amount of Ca^{++} mobilized in the terminal, thereby causing an increase in the amount of transmitter released onto the motor cell. Therefore, serotonin from the facilitating neuron causes an increase in the motor cell's response to the second neuron in the system.

CHAPTER 13

1. According to the World Health Organization, addiction is "a behavioral pattern of compulsive drug use, characterized by overwhelming involvement with the use of the drug, the securing of its supply, and a high tendency to relapse after withdrawal." Tolerance is a result of chronic use of some drugs. After a time, a greater dose is needed to produce the same result initially produced by a smaller dose. Dependence also results from chronic use. When removal of the drug results in a derangement of functioning, a disease called a withdrawal syndrome occurs. Dependence often accompanies tolerance, and many biomedical scientists use an operating definition of addiction that involves tolerance and dependence.

2. Many psychotropic drugs affect most cells in the body, as well as most cells in the central nervous system. Some of these many effects are more important than others, in terms of the user's motivation for taking the drug. Ethanol inhibits the locus ceruleus (LC) and also increases the effect of GABA at its primary (GABA-A) receptors. Both effects are depressant to the organism. Benzodiazepines and barbiturates also increase the effect of GABA at GABA-A receptors and are globally depressant. Barbiturates also inhibit mitochondrial metabolism, which is a globally depressant effect. Cocaine and amphetamines affect many functional proteins in the synapses of noradrenaline (NE), dopamine (DA), and acetylcholine (Ach), as well as other transmitters. Their major effects may result from inhibition of re-uptake of DA, which increases the activity of the DA. Opiates are direct agonists for the mu opioid receptor (and other opioid receptors) and have depressant effects in many places, especially in the LC.

3. Given the information in the answer to question 2, it is reasonable to focus

on GABA, NE, DA, and endogenous opioids (i.e., enkephalins, endorphins, and dynorphins) as the neurotransmitters most likely involved in the development of drug addiction.

CHAPTER 14

1. RQ, or respiratory quotient, is the ratio of the moles of CO_2 produced to the moles of O_2 consumed. This ratio can be determined for cells, organs, or whole organisms, more or less easily. The value of the RQ reflects the substrate(s) being metabolized (i.e., oxidized) by the preparation. The normal RQ of brain is 1.0, indicating relatively exclusive use of carbohydrate as an energy source. The term gluconeogenesis means synthesis of new glucose, and it is used to refer to the synthesis of glucose from the carbons of either amino acids or lactate. This occurs in liver or kidney, not in brain, and requires a source of energy as well as the carbon supply. The oxidation of fat often supplies the energy needed for gluconeogenesis, but the carbons from the fat cannot be a net source of carbons for glucose. The term ketone bodies refers to acetoacetate, beta-hydroxy butyrate, and acetone. These are made by liver from fats and can be used by many tissues, including brain, as an energy source. They cannot provide *all* the energy needed by the brain, however; the use of ketone bodies does not change the brain's requirement for glucose. Hypoglycemia is a relative term meaning abnormally low blood glucose. Anything below about 75 mg/dl (4.2 mM) could be called hypoglycemia, although clinical hypoglycemia is normally much lower than this.

2. The obligatory energy substrates for CNS metabolism are glucose and oxygen. The supplementary energy substrates are ketone bodies (the extent varying with the individual). Endogenous substrates, such as glycogen and pools of free amino acids, can be used in emergencies, but only glucose and related carbohydrates and ketone bodies can cross the blood–brain barrier in adequate amounts for energy production.

3. See the answer to question 2, above. Glycogen and pools of free amino acids are the energy reserve molecules. The pool of free amino acids is by far the larger, being able to support brain metabolism for half an hour or so when blood supplies fail.

4. Oxygen deficiency results in loss of consciousness in a few seconds and irreversible neuronal loss after a few minutes. Glucose deficiency results in confusion in minutes to an hour and brain damage after an hour or more, depending on other factors.

5. Cerebral blood flow (CBF) is predominantly regulated by the diameter of cerebral blood vessels: vasodilation increases CBF, vasoconstriction decreases it. Traditionally, pCO_2, pO_2, and pH were thought to be the major regulators of vasodilation. An elevation of pCO_2 or a decrease of pH causes vasodilation, and an increase of pO_2 causes vasoconstriction. These parameters fit with the metabolism of the tissue, in that metabolic products

increase CBF and a major metabolic substrate decreases it. Other factors that may also be involved (or even be more important) are adenosine (a degradation product of ATP, which may be found in all synaptic vesicles), ATP, and/or ADP. An additional factor recently shown to be important is nitric oxide (NO), and specific regulation by neuronal processes directly onto blood vessels may also occur.

CHAPTER 15

1. Negative feedback (NFB) and positive feed forward (PFF) are opposing regulatory mechanisms. NFB is the basic mechanism of stability, or homeostasis. For example, when the energy charge rises, ATP concentration is high. This inhibits those metabolic pathways that produce ATP, such as glycolysis and the citric acid cycle. PFF is necessary when it is desirable to override NFB and homeostasis, for example in learning. This kind of regulation is intrinsically unstable, so several inhibitory regulatory mechanisms must exist to control it.

2. The major source of acid in the CNS, as in the rest of the body, is carbon dioxide (CO_2), most of which is produced by the citric acid cycle in the mitochondrion. Nearly all the carbons of glucose, the major energy source for brain, leave the CNS as CO_2. Most of the carbons in amino acids and other molecules in brain also eventually leave as CO_2. Lactate is also produced by the brain and can be a significant source of acid, although the concentration of lactate may differ from the pH of the tissue.

3. GLUT1 and GLUT3 are two of several glucose transporters. Both are found in brain. GLUT1 is part of the blood–brain barrier and is partly affected by insulin. GLUT3 is a transporter in the neuronal membrane and is unaffected by insulin. GLUT3 probably functions to equalize glucose concentrations between extracellular fluid and neuronal cytoplasm; GLUT1 probably functions to increase glucose transport into the CNS from blood.

CHAPTER 16

1. The substantia nigra and the closely associated A9 and A10 nuclei are dopaminergic.

2. Although axons from the A9 and A10 nuclei are widespread, the cortex and the limbic system (amygdala, nucleus accumbens, cingulate gyrus, etc.) receive the major innervation. These are called the mesolimbic and mesocortical pathways.

3. The most important data supporting the dopamine hypothesis of schizophrenia arise from the clinical treatment of the disease by drugs that are antagonists (blockers) of dopamine receptors. Further, there is a rough

correlation between a drug's efficacy for treating schizophrenia and its potency as a DA receptor blocker. Newer generations of antipsychotic agents still appear to work primarily in DA synapses, but the specific mechanism of action is not entirely clear. There are other data that support this concept, for example the observation that a minority of patients treated for Parkinson's disease by increasing their DA activity show signs and symptoms similar to schizophrenia.

CHAPTER 17

1. GABA is usually considered to be the main transmitter involved in generalized anxiety, as it has relatively global activity within the CNS. The most common treatments for generalized anxiety use GABA antagonists at the GABA-A receptor.

2. Noradrenaline (NE) is often considered to be the main neurotransmitter determinant for panic disorders. However, as a second level transmitter, it works by modifying the underlying activity of amino acid transmitters (see the answer to question 1). Therefore, drugs that decrease GABA action can also be effective in treating other kinds of anxiety, such as panic disorders.

3. Benzodiazepines (BZPs) are secondary allosteric agonists of GABA-A receptors. This means that they have a binding site on the GABA-A receptor that is distinct from the GABA binding site. When BZPs are bound to their site, they modify the binding of GABA at its site, thereby increasing the effectiveness of GABA. This is a kind of secondary allosteric phenomenon, whereby one allosteric ligand affects the activity of another allosteric ligand. The natural, endogenous ligand for the BZP site is a peptide that probably has the opposite effect of BZPs and is thus anxiogenic.

4. Monoamineoxidase inhibitors (MAOIs) inhibit the enzyme (MAO) that destroys the activity of monoamine neurotransmitters such as dopamine (DA), noradrenaline (NE), and serotonin (5-HT). MAOIs therefore increase the concentrations of these transmitters, resulting in an increase in their synaptic activity. Tricyclic antidepressants (TCAs) are not as well understood. They are widely believed to function by inhibiting the re-uptake transporter for DA and NE. This action would result in an increase in activity for these synapses. However, the time course of clinical effectiveness of TCAs does not suggest this mechanism. It is possible that their mechanism of action is much more complex than this, possibly including receptor sensitivity modification, whereby the levels of postsynaptic receptor molecules are changed over time.

Glossary

A Alanine

acidosis The pathological condition of being too acidic, or lacking base. Normal pH of the bloodstream is considered to be about 7.4, with a range from 7.38 to 7.44. Any pH below 7.38 is acidotic. The normal pH in other body fluids may be different from that of blood, but the blood is usually monitored clinically.

action potential The term for a transient, all-or-nothing voltage change that conducts electrical current in neurons. It originates in the cell body of the neuron and is passed along its axon to the terminal. It has several different stages, the first of which is a movement of Na^+ ions into the neuron, producing a depolarization. This is followed by a movement of K^+ ions out of the neuron into the extracellular space, allowing restoration of the resting potential. After an action potential has passed, $Na^+ K^+$ ATPase restores both of these ions to their previous concentrations.

adenylyl cyclase The most recent name for the enzyme that makes $3', 5'$ cyclic adenosine monophosphate (cAMP) from ATP. It is an integral protein in the plasma membrane of many cells. Its active site and its substrate binding site are exposed to the cytoplasm of the cell, which is also where it produces the cAMP.

affective Referring to mental states of feeling

afferent In neurophysiology, moving toward the central nervous system, away from the periphery; centripetal

agonist In pharmacology, a molecule that binds to a receptor and affects it in the same way the endogenous activator does

alcohol 1. A carbon at an oxidation state in which it has one bond to an electronegative atom, such as oxygen or nitrogen. Methanol, CH_3OH, is a simple alcohol. 2. A term sometimes used as a synonym for ethyl alcohol, or ethanol (CH_3CH_2OH)

aldehyde A carbon at an oxidation level higher than that of an alcohol and lower than that of an acid. Most commonly, the carbon has two bonds to electronegative atom(s), such as oxygen or nitrogen. Formaldehyde, CH_2O, is a simple aldehyde.

alkyl A general term for a chain of carbon atoms attached to each other by saturated bonds

allosteric An adjective describing the process whereby a ligand affects a protein's function by modifying its three-dimensional structure as a result of binding to a specific regulatory site. An allosteric site is, by definition, at a distance on the molecule from its active site. An allosteric enzyme, for example, binds an inhibitor to an allosteric site, which results in a change in the structure of the active site that reduces the activity of the enzyme. An activator has the opposite effect. Ligand-activated ion channels (i.e., direct receptors) are allosteric protein complexes which, by binding the transmitter at a site distant from the ionophore, cause the channel to open.

amide   The name given a structure formed by combining the carboxyl group of an organic acid and an amino group. A water molecule is formed in the process. Amides are neutral and are relatively strong biological bonds.

amino acid   A class of biochemical molecules from which proteins are made. Each amino acid has one carboxyl and one amino (or imino) group, both of which are attached to the same carbon.

amino group   The $-NH_2$ group, usually bonded to a carbon. Amino groups are usually positively charged, as amines are basic ($-NH_2^+$).

amphoteric   Having opposite properties within the same molecule, e.g., both hydrophobic and hydrophilic properties (attraction to both aqueous and non-aqueous solvents); similarly, a molecule that has both acidic and basic groups

anabolism   That part of metabolism that involves the enzymatic synthesis of complex molecules. The term is most commonly applied to the synthesis of macromolecules, such as proteins, nucleic acids, complex carbohydrates, and complex lipids. Anabolism uses ATP as well as other nucleotide triphosphates.

anoxia   The total absence of oxygen

antagonist   In pharmacology, a molecule that nullifies the action of the primary, endogenous ligand. A drug or a toxin that binds to a receptor without activating it is an antagonist, because it blocks the usual ligand from binding. It therefore prevents the normal receptor response.

anterior   Toward the front, or belly, surface of the body, or toward the head

arachidonic acid   A naturally occurring fatty acid that contains twenty carbons and four double bonds (i.e., C20:4). It is the precursor for many biologically important regulators, including prostaglandins, prostacyclins, thromboxanes, and leukotrienes. Arachidonic acid cannot be fully synthesized by the human body, so either it or its precursors are essential dietary components.

associative learning   Learning whereby an organism acquires a relationship between two or more stimuli (classical conditioning) or between a stimulus and the organism's behavior (operant conditioning)

ataxia   Failure of muscular coordination

atherosclerosis   A narrowing of large and medium-sized arteries, caused by deposits of cholesterol and other lipids

autoantigen   A structural configuration of a molecule or molecules to which an organism can mount an immune response

autoimmune response   An immune response of an organism to some part of its own tissues

axo-axonic   Term for synapses in which the presynaptic portion comes from one neuron and the postsynaptic portion is provided by the presynaptic terminal of another synapse

axo-dendritic   Term for synapses in which the presynaptic portion is contributed by an axon and the postsynaptic portion is contributed by a dendrite

axo-somatic   Term for synapses in which the presynaptic portion is contributed by an axon and the postsynaptic part is contributed by a cell body, or soma

beta   1. The letter that identifies the second carbon in a sequence after the functional group. For example, the beta carbon of an amino acid is the third carbon, as the first carbon is part of the carboxyl functional group. 2. In stereochemistry, beta refers to attachments above the plane of a ring, such as in steroids or sugars. Alpha refers to constituents below the ring.

blood–brain barrier   A term that describes the observation that most molecules in the bloodstream do not pass into the central nervous system directly. This is more of a functional description than an anatomical one, as the anatomical basis for the barrier is not certain.

brainstem   Anatomical structure composed of the medulla, pons and cerebellum, and midbrain. The brainstem receives sensory information from cranial structures and controls the muscles of the head. It carries information reversibly between the spinal cord and the hemispheres. It also contains the parts of the CNS that control arousal.

C   Cysteine

calmodulin (CM)   A low-molecular-weight (about 17,000), highly conserved protein that contains four binding sites for calcium. Calmodulin with one or more calciums bound to it is an allosteric activator of many proteins.

cAMP $3', 5'$ cyclic adenosine monophosphate. An allosteric regulator produced by adenylyl cyclase in response to the activation of many receptors. It should not be confused with AMP, adenosine monophosphate, which is a similar molecule without the cyclic ring structure. AMP's biochemical activities are quite distinct from those of cAMP.

carboxyl group   A carbon at the oxidation level of an organic acid, above that of an aldehyde. In biology, the carbon most commonly has three bonds to an electronegative atom, such as oxygen or nitrogen.

catabolism   The part of metabolism that involves the enzymatic degradation of biological molecules into smaller parts, progressing to total combustion to final end products such as carbon dioxide, urea, and water. Catabolism normally produces ATP, which is then available for anabolism and other processes.

catalytic   An adjective describing a substance that can increase the speed of a chemical reaction without itself being consumed in the reaction. Enzymes are biological catalysts. A catalytic coenzyme, or cofactor, is a non-protein molecule that is required for the full catalysis of a reaction and is also not consumed in the reaction.

ceramide   A general term for a molecule that contains a fatty acid attached in amide linkage to a sphingosine. The name ceramide is used regardless of the particular fatty acid involved and regardless of the chain length or degree of unsaturation of the sphingosine.

cerebroside   A glycolipid containing a sphingosine and a fatty acid (a ceramide) and a single sugar attached to the first carbon of the sphingosine. The most common cerebroside in normal brain contains galactose as the sugar residue.

cerebrospinal fluid (CSF)   A fluid that fills the ventricles of the brain and surrounding spaces. It flows continuously, arising in the interior of the brain and ending in the bloodstream.

cGMP $3', 5'$ cyclic guanosine monophosphate; an allosteric regulator of protein function similar to cAMP, but less widespread

cholesterol An important biological molecule found predominantly in cell membranes, where it is present in the largest molar amount of any molecule. Cholesterol is also found in blood lipoproteins and in pathological deposits in skin and other tissues.

choline One of the most fundamental biochemical nitrogen-containing molecules. Choline is not found in large quantity as a separate molecule, but is an important constituent of other important molecules. Phosphatidyl choline (also called lecithin) is one of the major phospholipids in biology. Choline is also an important component of sphingomyelin, an important sphingolipid, and of acetyl choline, an important neurotransmitter.

$$HO-CH_2CH_2-\overset{\overset{\displaystyle CH_3}{|}}{\underset{\underset{\displaystyle CH_3}{|}}{\overset{+}{N}}}-CH_3$$

cirrhosis Interstitial inflammation, especially of the liver. Cirrhotic livers often decrease in size, becoming fibrous tissue. Many normal liver functions are lost as a result of cirrhosis.

cis In organic chemistry, a term referring to a configuration in which constituents are on the same side of a carbon-carbon double bond (see also *trans*). A *cis* double bond within an alkyl chain has two hydrogens on the same side:

$$R-\overset{\overset{\displaystyle H}{|}}{C}=\overset{\overset{\displaystyle H}{|}}{C}-R$$

citric acid cycle The metabolic pathway in mitochondria that oxidizes most of the carbons in foodstuffs to carbon dioxide (CO_2); also known as the tricarboxylic acid (TCA) cycle or the Krebs' cycle

cloning In biochemistry, a process in which a single portion of DNA, or the DNA of a single cell, is replicated

CNS The central nervous system, consisting of both the brain and the spinal cord

coenzyme A cofactor for an enzyme, required for the enzymatic reaction. Coenzymes that are needed in amounts equal to the amounts of the substrates of the reaction are stoichiometric cofactors. Coenzymes that are needed only on a one-to-one basis with the enzyme are catalytic cofactors.

coenzyme A The name given to a particular stoichiometric coenzyme that contains the vitamin pantothenic acid and is used in the metabolism of acyl groups.

cofactor A general term for a molecule that must be present for another molecule to function

coma A state of unconsciousness from which the person cannot be aroused

conditioned stimulus (CS) In classical, Pavlovian conditioning, a stimulus that does not produce the effect of the unconditioned stimulus (UCS) in an organism, but that can be made to do so. In the process of conditioning (i.e., pairing the CS and the UCS in specific ways), the CS comes to produce the same effect as the UCS.

contralateral Referring to the opposite side (contrasted to ypsilateral, or ipsilateral). Many nervous system pathways cross the midline, moving from one side to the contralateral side. Most functions in the brain are duplicated, being represented in the same anatomical structure on both sides of the brain. An activity in one location is often paired with similar activity on the contralateral side. Many functions are represented in only one hemisphere, however.

cortex   The outer layer of the brain (the Latin word means "bark"), typically several layers of cells deep. The convoluted surface features of the human brain give the cortex a very large surface area. About half of all human neurons are in the cortex of the cerebral hemispheres.

cyclic AMP   *See* cAMP

cyclic GMP   *See* cGMP

D   Aspartate, or aspartic acid

DAG   Diacyl glycerol, a glycerol moiety with two fatty acids attached to its number 1 and 2 carbons, in ester linkage. Because the fatty acids may vary, diacyl glycerol is a polydisperse molecule. DAGs, when produced at the surface between the cytoplasm of a cell and its plasma membrane, are allosteric activators of protein kinase C.

declarative memory   The product of learning that involves cognition. Its formation requires such brain structures as the hippocampus and/or the amygdala.

dementia   A general term for loss or severe deterioration of mentation, or mind. The term dementia is commonly applied to adults.

dependence   In neuropharmacology, a state in which a person requires chronic doses of a drug to prevent the onset of a withdrawal sickness

depolarization   Removing the polarity of a nerve cell's membrane. If the depolarization is great enough, an action potential will be produced. The resting potential of a neuron is about -70 mV; therefore, a depolarization is a movement in a positive direction.

depression   In psychiatry, an absence of hope; severe dejection. It is commonly accompanied by a decrease in many physiological functions as well as mental ones.

diacyl glycerol   *See* DAG

digested   In biochemistry, a term that normally means the same as "hydrolyzed." The digestive process in the gut involves the hydrolysis of foodstuffs.

dipeptide   A misnomer, used to indicate a molecule with two amino acids joined by a single peptide (amide) bond. Similarly, a tripeptide has three amino acids and two peptide bonds.

disaccharide   A molecule that contains two sugar residues. Table sugar is a disaccharide of glucose and fructose.

disinhibition   The process of generating a stimulation by removing a previous inhibition. The concept applies at the molecular, cellular, organ system, and organism levels.

dorsal   Toward the back, or posterior

E   Glutamate, or glutamic acid

edema   Excessive accumulation of fluid in intercellular or intracellular spaces. Intracellular edema is more toxic.

effector   An agent that causes a change. The term is used in biochemistry in describing allosterically regulated protein complexes, wherein an effector can be either positive or negative (i.e., stimulatory or inhibitory). An allosteric effector is not directly involved in the activity of the regulated complex; it only modifies the degree of activity.

efferent   In neurophysiology, moving away from the central nervous system, toward the periphery; centrifugal

eicosanoids   A general term for those classes of biologically active lipid molecules made from arachidonic acid (C20:4). These include prostaglandins, prostacyclins, thromboxanes, and leukotrienes.

endoplasmic reticulum (ER)   The network of membrane-bound channels in the interior of a cell that is surrounded by cytoplasm. The interior, or lumen, of the ER is connected to the Golgi apparatus. Smooth endoplasmic reticulum (SER) is the site of synthesis of many lipids. Rough endoplasmic reticulum (RER) is the site of protein synthesis.

energy charge (EC)   The ratio of adenine nucleotides that is the central allosteric regulator of metabolism. It is defined as

$$EC = \frac{(ATP) + 1/2\,(ADP)}{(ATP) + (ADP) + (AMP)}$$

A high energy charge favors anabolism; a low energy charge favors catabolism.

engram   The traces of a memory stored in the brain; the physical end product of learning

epitope   A specific antigenic site. This is the term for the specific site to which an antibody or an immune cell binds.

essential   In biochemistry, the adjective used to refer to molecules that are *dietary* essentials. These are necessary for metabolism and cannot be synthesized within the body. All biological molecules present in the body are, of course, essential for healthy function, but those that can be synthesized within the body are called non-essential.

ester   The product of the combination of an acid and an alcohol, with the loss of water

ether   A molecule made by replacing the two hydrogens of a water molecule with alkyl groups

etiology   The study of causes; the specific cause or origin of a disease

F   Phenylalanine

free radical   A chemical structure that contains at least one unpaired electron. Many free radicals are highly reactive and can start chain reactions that can be destructive to cells. Some free radicals (e.g., vitamin E) are stable and can stop chain reactions and prevent further injury.

G   Glycine

G protein   Proteins that bind GTP. They are also GTPases, hydrolyzing the GTP to GDP and P.

ganglioside   The most structurally complex class of glycolipids. A ganglioside, by definition, contains one or more sialic acid (N-acetyl neuraminic acid) residues and a ceramide. Gangliosides also contain one or more sugar residues.

Gi   A G protein that produces an inhibitory effect on another molecule while it is bound to a GTP

gluconeogenesis The metabolic pathway that synthesizes glucose from other molecules. The most common source of carbons in the newly synthesized glucose is either amino acids or lactic acid. Gluconeogenesis requires energy, commonly supplied by the oxidation of fats.

glutathione A tripeptide found in high concentration in the cytoplasm of most cells. It contains residues of glutamate, cysteine, and glycine. The sulfhydryl group of the cysteine plays an important role in preventing the oxidation of cytoplasmic contents.

glyco- A prefix (from the Greek word meaning "sweet") used to designate molecules containing sugar residues. Glycolipids and glycoproteins are classes of molecules modified by the addition of sugars.

glycoconjugates The general term for both lipids and proteins with carbohydrates attached

glycoprotein Proteins to which carbohydrate residues have been attached

glycosidase An enzyme that hydrolyzes a sugar residue from a larger molecule

glycosylation The enzymatic addition of a sugar residue to a molecule. The term is most commonly used to refer to the construction of glycoproteins and glycolipids.

gray matter Clusters of neuronal cell bodies within the central nervous system. Axons, individually or in bundles, extend from regions of gray matter to other parts of the nervous system. Gray matter is distinct from white matter, which is regions of axons and their myelin sheaths.

Gs A G protein that produces a stimulatory effect on another molecule while bound to a GTP

H Histidine

habituation The simplest kind of learning, in which a stimulus produces less of a response after repetition

hepatitis Inflammation of the liver

heptahelical Having seven helices; a general term for the rhodospin family of receptors. All of these have seven alpha helices that traverse the plasma membrane; all also with G proteins.

hippocampus A seahorse-shaped portion of the temporal lobe of the brain, next to the lateral ventricles. The hippocampus is topologically a part of the cortex but is buried deep within the brain. It is an important part of the limbic system and is believed to be necessary for the learning of spatial memories.

homeostasis In normal physiology, the tendency toward stability, which is brought about by regulatory mechanisms that return physiology to normal after a perturbation. Negative feedback (NFB) is the most common regulatory mechanism for achieving homeostasis.

homotropic Word used to describe a regulatory change that is opposite in direction to that of homeostasis; in other words, a regulatory response that is in the same direction as the perturbation. (For example, when the hippocampus is stimulated in a particular way, it becomes "set" to a higher response to successive stimulation.) Positive feed forward (PFF) is an example of homotropic regulation.

hydrolase An enzyme that catalyzes a hydrolysis

hydrolysis The process of breaking a chemical bond by adding a molecule of water to it. The hydroxyl group of the water appears in one product and the remaining hydrogen in the other.

hydrophilic Having an affinity for water; the term for molecules or parts of molecules that form associations with water molecules. Carbohydrates and some amino acid side chains (e.g., E, D, Q, N, K, R) are strongly hydrophilic.

hydrophobic Water-avoiding; the term for molecules or parts of molecules that are repelled by water and therefore do not dissolve in it. Fatty acids and some amino acid side chains (e.g., L, V, I, F) are hydrophobic.

hydroxyl 1. An $-OH$ group attached to something else. This is called a hydroxyl group. The addition of this group to reduced carbon makes it an alcohol. 2. A hydroxyl molecule is $\cdot OH$, which is a highly reactive (and toxic) free radical.

hyperemesis Excessive vomiting

hyperpolarization The inhibition of a neuron's firing by the reduction of its resting membrane potential below the resting potential; the opposite of depolarization

hypertrophy The morbid enlargement of an organ or a part of an organ, due to an increase in the size of constituent cells

hypoglycemia Too little blood sugar. Normal blood sugar is between 4.2 mM and 5.8 mM (75 to 105 mg/dl). Any lower value is hypoglycemia.

hypoxia Low or inadequate oxygen content

I Isoleucine

inositol trisphosphate (IP3) Most commonly, inositol 1,4,5 trisphosphate, a second messenger. Inositol (most commonly *myo*inositol in biology) is a cyclic derivative of glucose containing six carbons, each of which has a hydroxyl group. There are many different possible inositol trisphosphates, but the 1,4,5 isomer is the most active.

integral In biochemistry, the term for a protein that is incorporated into a membrane rather than attached to one of its surfaces. Such a protein must have at least one part of its sequence embedded within the hydrophobic part of the membrane.

interneuron Any neuron in a sequence that is between the primary afferent and the final motor neuron. The term is most commonly used for neurons with short axons that connect two or more neurons that are near each other.

interstitial Referring to the spaces, or gaps, in a tissue; commonly used to refer to the extracellular structures in a tissue

ionophore The aperture of an ion channel, that part of the channel that allows ions to pass from one side of the membrane to the other. Ion channels are composed of more than one polypeptide subunit, usually with each subunit contributing one transmembrane segment to make the channel. Many channels are selective, in that only certain ions are allowed to pass.

IP3 *See* inositol trisphosphate

ipsilateral Pertaining to the same side; often used in describing functions in the brain and central nervous system

ischemia Deficiency of blood supply

isoelectric Showing no variation in electric potential; in neurology, the absence of measurable brain electrical activity (i.e., lack of physiological evidence of action potentials)

isoenzyme *See* isozyme

isoprenyl group A group named after isoprene, a five-carbon intermediate in the synthesis of lipids such as steroids. Isoprenoids are various multiples of this five-carbon unit. Isoprenyl groups of various kinds are found covalently attached to regulatory sites of many proteins.

isozyme One of several different forms of an enzyme that catalyze the same reaction. Different isozymes may have strikingly different kinetic, physical, chemical, or immunological properties.

K Lysine

K_D Affinity constant. Although it can be described mathematically in several ways, basically K_D is that concentration of an agent (e.g., a drug) that gives half its maximal effect. It therefore is expressed as units of concentration. The affinity constant is probably best used for those agents that are not changed by the act of binding. Examples are drugs, hormones and/or transmitters binding to receptors, or allosteric effectors binding to enzymes. The lower the affinity constant, the tighter the binding.

ketose A sugar that contains a ketone group. In biochemistry, the ketone group is most commonly on the second carbon. The ketone group has the same oxidation level as an aldehyde group.

Km Michaelis constant. Although it has several mathematical definitions, it is the concentration of substrate that provides half of the maximal velocity of an enzyme reaction. It is expressed in units of concentration. It is most often used for molecules that are changed as a result of the binding, as is the case for a substrate's binding an enzyme. The lower the Km, the tighter the binding.

L Leucine

leukocytes (or leucocytes) Colorless blood cells of many types. Leukocytes are generally protective and many are a part of the immune system.

ligand A general term for a molecule that binds to a receptor. Most commonly, a ligand is a small molecule that binds to a macromolecule.

limbic system A group of brain structures that are phylogenetically old and are thought to be important in olfaction, emotion, and behavior

lysosomes Cellular organelles, each of which contains a large number of different hydrolases

M Methionine

mania A mental state characterized by elation, expansiveness, overtalkativeness, wild flights of ideas, and increased motor activity

manic-depressive disorder A mental disorder that can be characterized either by severe depression (unipolar) or by both mania and depression (bipolar)

mesencephalon The midbrain. It lies below the cerebral hemispheres and is a part of the brainstem

Michaelis constant *See* Km

midbrain *See* mesencephalon

moiety Chemical term for a portion of a molecule that can be considered to have chemical properties of its own

monodisperse A term used to refer to a substance in which every molecule is identical to every other. Crystals of small molecules and of many proteins are monodisperse.

motor   Referring to movement. A nerve that activates a muscle is a motor nerve.

muscarinic   One class of acetylcholine receptors. The alkaloid muscarine is an agonist for these receptors. They are the predominant class of acetylcholine receptor in brain, belonging to the heptahelical family of receptors.

myelin   The multiple layers of compacted, lipid-filled membranes that surround and insulate axons

N   Asparagine

N-acetyl neuraminic acid (NANA)   *See* sialic acid

NANA   N-acetyl neuraminic acid; *see* sialic acid

negative feedback (NFB)   The process in which one or more of the products of a metabolic pathway inhibits the pathway

neuraminidase   An enzyme that hydrolyzes N-acetyl neuraminic acid from its glycosidic attachments; also called sialidase

nicotinic   One class of acetylcholine receptors. The alkaloid nicotine is an agonist for these receptors. Nicotinic receptors are direct receptors and are rapid acting.

nitric oxide (NO)   A small molecule that is a biological regulator. It is made from arginine and oxygen by nitric oxide synthetase (NOS) and has both toxic and protective properties in cells, depending on the circumstances. There are other forms of nitrogen monoxides, but nitric oxide refers to the free radical.

NO   *See* nitric oxide

non-associative learning   The simplest kind of learning, either habituation or sensitization

non-essential   In biochemistry, a term for molecules that the organism can synthesize from small molecule precursors. Non-essential molecules are necessary for metabolism, but they are not essential components of the organism's diet.

5′-nucleotidase   An enzyme that hydrolyzes the phosphate group (attached to the fifth carbon of the ribose) from a nucleotide. The products are commonly a phosphate group and a nucleoside.

nucleus (pl. nuclei)   1. A membrane-bound cellular organelle containing the cell's DNA (i.e., genetic material). 2. In the CNS, a cluster of neuronal perikarya

oocytes   Immature egg cells

P   Proline

PAM   Peptidyl glycine alpha-amidating monooxygenase. An enzyme in brain that oxidizes the carbons of a C-terminal glycine on a peptide, leaving an amide group on the penultimate amino acid

penumbra   In neurology, the area surrounding the focal site of injury in the CNS and secondarily affected by the injury

peptidase   An enzyme that hydrolyzes one or more bonds in a peptide

peptide bonds   Amide bonds joining the alpha carboxyl group of one amino acid to the alpha amino group of another, with a loss of a water molecule

peptidergic   Refers to synapses in which a peptide is the transmitter

peptides   Unbranched sequences of amino acids connected by peptide bonds. The term is commonly reserved for peptides smaller than proteins, which are called polypeptides.

peptidyl glycine alpha-amidating monooxygenase *See* PAM

perikaryon (pl. perikarya) The cell body of a neuron, as opposed to the processes, such as axons, dendrites, etc.

peripheral nervous system *See* PNS

PFF *See* positive feed forward

photon A particle, or quantum, of radiant energy. The wavelength of a photon reflects its energy content.

phylogenetic Referring to the complete developmental (i.e., evolutionary) history of a group of organisms

PLP A coenzyme that is made from vitamin B_6, or pyridoxine. It is used by most enzymes that metabolize substituents on the number 2 (i.e., alpha) carbon of amino acids.

PNS Peripheral nervous system; the extensive network of nerves connecting the central nervous system to the rest of the body

polydisperse Substances that are not exactly homogeneous, in which small variations of structure exist from one molecule to another, but wherein all molecules have the same overall chemical properties; most obviously true of lipids and complex carbohydrates

polygenetic Capable of arising in many different ways. In medicine, the term is used to describe a disease that can be caused by several different mechanisms. For example, gout (gouty arthritis), resulting from excess uric acid in blood, can be caused by deficiencies of some enzymes, excess activity of other enzymes, or an inadequacy of secretion of uric acid into the urine.

polygenic Requiring multiple genes. A polygenic biological characteristic (e.g., height) is one that requires the interaction of several different genes rather than the expression of a single gene (as does skin color, for example).

POMC Proopiomelanocortin; the name of a polypeptide precursor for several neuropeptides, including beta endorphin, gamma melanocyte stimulating hormone (MSH), and adrenocorticotropin (ACTH). It is made by cells in the pituitary and hypothalamus.

positive feed forward (PFF) A regulatory response in which an enhanced stimulus results in a long-term increase in the response of the system to subsequent stimuli. PFF is in the opposite direction from NFB, or homeostatic regulation.

post-transcriptional Occurring after transcription, which is the process of making RNA molecules in accordance with the DNA sequence in genes

post-translational modifications Changes in the structure of a protein that occur after it has been synthesized (protein synthesis is called translation); specifically, chemical changes made to the side chains of amino acids. The addition of one or more phosphate residues or sugar residues is a common post-translational modification. Such changes modify the function of the protein.

preproproteins General designation for proproteins that are synthesized with a "signal" peptide sequence. The signal sequence assists the polypeptide in crossing membranes. The signal sequence is often near the N-terminal part of the molecule.

primary structure In biochemistry, the sequence of nucleotides in nucleic acids or of amino acids in proteins. Proteins' amino acid sequences are numbered starting from the N-terminus; nucleic acids start from the 5′ terminus. Macromolecules have additional levels of structure: secondary, tertiary, etc.

proopiomelanocortin *See* POMC

proproteins General designation for protein precursors from which smaller, biologically active peptides or proteins are produced by hydrolysis

prostaglandins A class of fatty acids containing twenty carbons and various numbers of double bonds, carbonyl groups, or hydroxyl groups, that are made from arachidonic acid. Prostaglandins are important biological regulators with properties similar to hormones.

psychosis A generic term for the most severe mental disorders. Schizophrenia and manic-depressive psychosis account for the bulk of psychoses.

psychotropic Affecting the mind

pyridoxal phosphate *See* PLP

Q Glutamine

quaternary structure In biochemistry, a structure created by combining several individual macromolecules in a specific way. For example, hemoglobin is composed of four separate polypeptides, of two different kinds. Receptors for hormones and transmitters are complexes of four or more individual polypeptides.

R Arginine

reflexive memory The product of a type of simple learning that has an automatic quality about it. Its acquisition is based on repetition and is not dependent on awareness, cognition, or consciousness; sometimes called habit

residue A chemical group that is a part of a larger molecule but that can be freed by hydrolysis. Therefore, a residue of a substance differs from the free substance by the molecular weight of one water molecule. For example, proteins contain residues of amino acids.

S Serine

saccharide *See* sugar

S-adenosyl methionine *See* SAM

saltatory Leaping or dancing; used to describe the conduction of an action potential down an axon as it "jumps" from node to node

SAM S-adenosyl methionine; a derivative of the amino acid methionine containing a metabolically active methyl group. It is the most common source of methyl groups that are enzymatically added to lipids and neurotransmitters.

satiety The feeling of being satisfied, of no longer desiring food

saturated 1. In enzymology, referring to an enzyme's being fully bound to substrate. At saturation, the enzyme is catalyzing its reaction at maximum velocity. 2. In organic chemistry, saturated compounds are those in which all carbon valences, other than single carbon-carbon bonds, are filled with hydrogen.

Schiff base A covalent linkage between an aldehyde group and an amino group, formed with the loss of a water molecule. Schiff bases form readily and hydrolyze just as readily, often without enzymes. Schiff bases are a part of the mechanism of action of many enzymes that use pyridoxal phosphate (PLP) as a cofactor.

secondary structure In biochemistry, the hydrogen-bonded first layer of three-dimensional structure superimposed on primary structure. Secondary structure arises from interactions among residues that are non-adjacent but close to each other. For example, the secondary structure of a protein is formed by hydrogen bonds among the atoms of the peptide bonds in the primary sequence. These hydrogen bonds are typically formed between residues three or four positions distant from each other.

sensitization (potentiation)   A kind of non-associative learning in which one stimulus increases the response to another. Sensitization prevents habituation and can reverse it.

sensory   Referring to sensation. A nerve that carries information from the periphery to the central nervous system is sensory.

sequencing   In biochemistry, the process of determining the primary structure of nucleic acids or proteins. This requires determining the exact location, within the sequence, of each nucleotide or amino acid.

sialic acid (also called NANA, or N-acetyl neuraminic acid)   A complex, nine-carbon sugar derivative that is common on terminal positions of glycoconjugates. (The structure is given in Chapter 2 on page 18.) It carries a negative charge at neutral pH and is most commonly found on the outermost portions of cells.

sialidase   An enzyme specific for the hydrolysis of sialic acid residues; also called neuraminidase

sphingomyelin   A common sphingolipid, found in most membranes in the body. It is composed of a ceramide bound to phosphoryl choline.

sphingosine   A long-chain fatty base, which forms the backbone of the class of molecules called sphingolipids. These include sphingomyelin, cerebrosides, sulfatides, gangliosides, and others. Sphingolipids are found in high concentration in nervous tissue.

spontaneous   1. In physical chemistry, the term for a reaction that can proceed, i.e., a possible reaction. 2. In biochemistry, the term for a reaction that is non-enzymatic, i.e., that proceeds by itself whenever the reactants are present in sufficient quantity

stoichiometric   Referring to the ratios of molecules involved in a chemical reaction. A stoichiometric cofactor in an enzymatic reaction is one that is treated as a substrate by the enzyme.

sugar   A molecule containing three or more carbons, all but one of which are alcohols. The non-alcohol carbon is at the aldehyde level of oxidation (i.e., an aldehyde or a ketone); also called a saccharide

symport   The movement of two molecules simultaneously in the same direction

symporter   A molecule that transports two substances simultaneously across membranes in the same direction. For example, most amino acids and sugars are translocated across membranes by a symporter requiring a Na^+ ion in conjunction with the amino acid or sugar. Both the Na^+ ion and the other molecule are transported into the cytoplasm.

T   Threonine

TCA cycle   *See* citric acid cycle

tertiary structure   In biochemistry, the three-dimensional conformation of a macromolecule, formed by interactions among residues at some distance from each other in the primary sequence

tolerance In pharmacology, a decreased susceptibility to a drug's effects as a result of its chronic use

trans In chemistry, a term that indicates that constituents are located on opposite sides of a carbon-carbon double bond; opposed to *cis*, which indicates that the constituents are located on the same side

```
        H
        |
R — C = C — R
        |
        H
```

transcription In biochemistry, the synthesis of messenger RNA from the information in one or more genes (i.e., DNA). The process is called transcription because the information is encoded in similar chemical groups in the two molecules and thus is simply copied from the DNA to the RNA.

translation In biochemistry, the synthesis of protein from the information in RNA. Since the information for the molecular structure is transferred from a nucleic acid to a protein, it is being "translated" from one language to another.

trophic (or tropic) Traditionally, a term referring to nutrition. Currently the term refers to affinity. A psychotropic drug is one that specifically affects the psyche, or mind.

unconditioned stimulus (UCS) In classical conditioning, a stimulus that produces an overt, quantifiable response in the organism being studied

unsaturated In organic chemistry, compounds containing two or more carbon atoms joined by double or triple bonds; a molecule to which various atoms, such as hydrogen, can be added (not substituted)

V Valine

ventricle A cavity or chamber. Within the CNS there is a system of ventricles that interconnect and are filled with continuously flowing cerebrospinal fluid.

W Tryptophan

white matter The portions of the CNS, visibly whiter than the rest, that contain multiple axons surrounded by myelin sheaths

Xenopus laevis A species of frog whose eggs are commonly used for research

Y Tyrosine

INDEX